Widad A. Abd Al-Behadili
Mohamed Abdel-Raheem

Medicinal Plants: Phytochemical Constituents & Therapeutic Potentials

AF784162

Widad A. Abd Al-Behadili
Mohamed Abdel-Raheem

Medicinal Plants: Phytochemical Constituents & Therapeutic Potentials

Noor Publishing

Imprint
Any brand names and product names mentioned in this book are subject to trademark, brand or patent protection and are trademarks or registered trademarks of their respective holders. The use of brand names, product names, common names, trade names, product descriptions etc. even without a particular marking in this work is in no way to be construed to mean that such names may be regarded as unrestricted in respect of trademark and brand protection legislation and could thus be used by anyone.

Cover image: www.ingimage.com

Publisher:
Noor Publishing
is a trademark of
Dodo Books Indian Ocean Ltd. and OmniScriptum S.R.L publishing group

120 High Road, East Finchley, London, N2 9ED, United Kingdom
Str. Armeneasca 28/1, office 1, Chisinau MD-2012, Republic of Moldova, Europe
Managing Directors: Ieva Konstantinova, Victoria Ursu
info@omniscriptum.com

Printed at: see last page
ISBN: 978-620-9-53352-5

Medicinal Plants: Phytochemical Constituents & Therapeutic Potentials

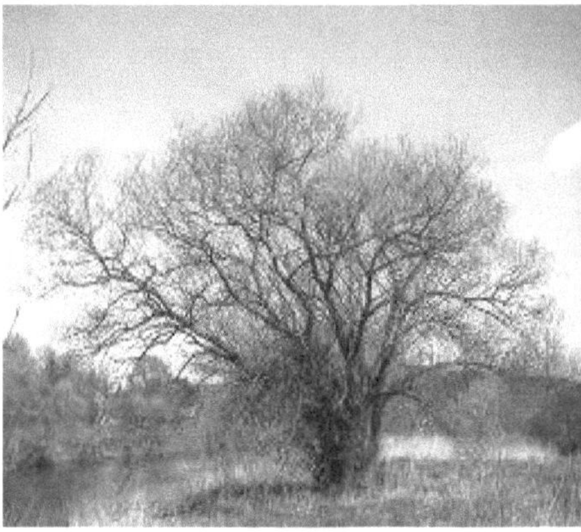

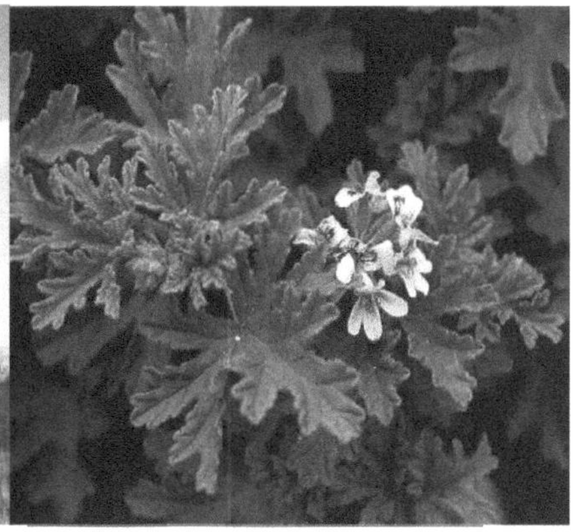

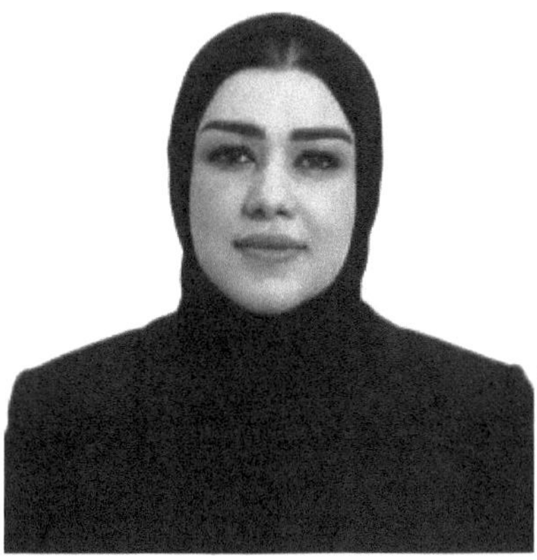

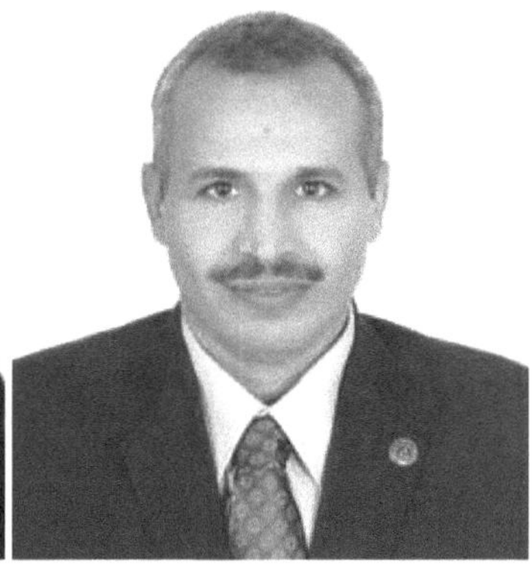

By

Assist. Prof. Dr. Widad A. Abd Al-Behadili

Prof. Dr. Mohamed Abdel-Raheem

(2026)

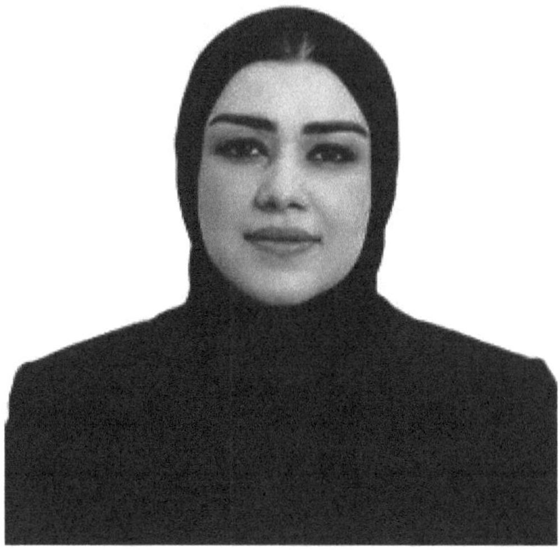

Assist. Prof. Dr. Widad A. Abd Al-Behadili

Department of Pharmacognosy and Medicinal Plants, College of Pharmacy, University of Misan, Maysan, Iraq.

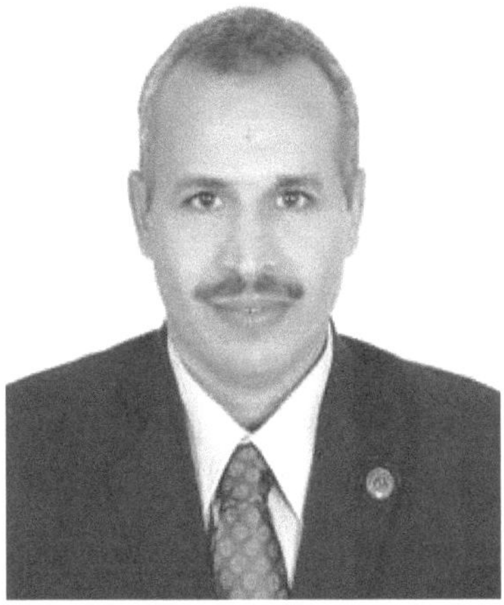

Prof. Dr. Mohamed Abdel-Raheem Ali Abdel-Raheem

Professor of Biological Control

Pests & Plant Protection Department

Agricultural and Biological Research Institute

National Research Centre.

Content list

Introduction

Angiogenesis, fibrosis, tissue damage, and altered cellular metabolism are all consequences of prolonged exposure to inflammatory mediators that may have an impact on overall health. Additionally, it is a major risk factor for a number of diseases, including as arthritis, diabetes, cancer, heart disease, and stroke.

As a result, scientists must investigate novel, secure, and efficient alternative treatments for persistent inflammation [**1-3**].

Because of their great diversity, plant-based phytochemicals are becoming cutting-edge tools for preventing chronic diseases—treating a broad spectrum of inflammatory medical conditions, including cancer, cardiovascular disease, autoimmune disorders, and neurological disorders—and they have also proven themselves to be excellent candidates for the creation of new drugs. The possibility of phytochemical constituents found in medicinal plants is under research as a new and promising therapy choice for chronic inflammation [**4-6**].

These naturally derived compounds have a great safety record and several anti-inflammatory properties. By accepting the great diversity of phytochemicals found in medicinal plants, which would eventually improve the health of many individuals worldwide, it may be possible to find new and successful therapies for chronic inflammatory diseases.

Traditional Chinese medicine (TCM) and herbal medications have effectively used a multifaceted medical strategy. [**7-8**]

The merger of conventional molecular biological research, analysis of extensive biological data, and application of artificial intelligence technology has led to a rapid evolution in efforts to improve understanding of the disease.

Examining the polypharmacological effects of several ingredients requires a substantial investment of time and money, which is usually spent on traditional research. Consequently, a more thorough approach is required in order to gain a deep comprehension of the illness and create better treatments. Because of the wide range of components found in natural goods, maintaining quality control to ensure constant efficacy is still difficult, despite the positive results and numerous research initiatives. Assessing the chemical makeup and purity of medications or herbal remedies is included in chemical quality control. [**9-11**]. Chemical quality control has disadvantages even though it is essential for confirming the efficacy and safety of medications. By integrating chemical and biological quality control, these limitations can be overcome. By identifying possible contaminants that can evade chemical examination and providing a more accurate evaluation of the product's effects, using in vitro or in vivo methods to analyze the biological activity of a medication or herbal remedy enhances biological quality control.

Biological quality control is a helpful supplement to chemical quality control to guarantee the efficacy and safety of herbal medicines and drugs. The use of phytochemicals for treating conditions associated with inflammation is under study in this Special Issue, which aims to improve anti-inflammatory power and induce reactions within innate immune systems that regulate genetic stability by carefully mixing chemicals that target various pathways. These strategies might help to improve the chances of discovering a therapy of clinical importance. **[12].** Infections, inflammation, diabetes mellitus, cancer, cardiovascular diseases and gastrointestinal disorders remain prominent factors contributing to global mortality and morbidity of particular concern are the severe complications associated with chronic illnesses that can greatly diminish quality of life. The effectiveness of the synthetic drugs currently on the market for treating these conditions is frequently limited by their side effects. These restrictions include hypersensitivity reactions, possible drug interactions, and unfavorable side effects. Furthermore, a sizable section of the world's population has difficulty affording and readily obtaining synthetic medications. [**12- 22**].

Since medicinal plants are typically regarded as safer, more accessible, and less expensive than synthetic medications, ethnomedicine has long valued them as therapeutic agents. According to the World Health Organization (WHO), traditional plant-based medicines continue to provide primary medical care for more than 80% of people worldwide. In recent years, medicinal plants have drawn more attention globally as potential alternatives to synthetic medications.

In contrast to synthetic drugs, which are typically based on a single active chemical compound, plant-based medicines contain a variety of phytoconstituents, such as flavonoids, alkaloids, polyphenols, and terpenoids. Increasing their therapeutic efficacy, these phytochemicals have been shown to interact with multiple biological targets simultaneously to produce their pharmacological effects. Findings that certain phytoconstituents in a plant extract can boost the bioactivity of others through a process known as "synergism" provide more proof in favor of the use of medicinal plants. **[23- 25].**

Usage of botanical substances in traditional forms of healthcare

The utilisation of botanical resources in treating and prevention of disease in various cultural set ups is known as ethnomedicine. Throughout human evolutionary history, medicinal flora has been used, particularly the people in rural and remote areas, as part of native medical knowledge, used therapeutic system and is mostly practiced in India although it has been maintained in some other countries of Southeast Asia like Bangladesh, Sri Lanka, Nepal, and Pakistan. In India, there are over twenty thousand formally recognised medicinal flora **[26- 28].**

Unani medicine- sometimes known as Greco-Arabian or Persian system- is a holistic system of healing which developed out of the ancient Greek medicine of Hippocrates and Galen, and then was enhanced and standardised by Arab and Persian thinkers in the Middle Ages. The essence of it is a humoral theory which moderates the four fluids of the body (blood, phlegm, yellow bile, black bile) by means of the diet, herbs, massage, and lifestyle.

On introducing it to India in the medieval era, it was mixed with the medical knowledge of the Indians, and evolved into a unique Indian Unani form of practice, which continues to be taught in Indian universities and practiced in clinics throughout the sub-continent. Unani is today a recognized conventional medical system by the World Health Organization and has still remained commonly used in most Arabic and Asian nations, providing an integrated approach to health to complement modern medicine. **[29- 31].**

TCM, with more than 2000 years of used in disease therapy from China, Japan, and other Eastern and Southeastern countries with the same cultural background.

Traditional Chinese Medicine (TCM) continues to be an essential element of the contemporary Chinese healthcare system and is increasingly gaining global recognition as a complementary and alternative form of healthcare. The utilization of medicinal plants in TCM encompasses a diverse array of species **[32, 33].** Remaining pertinent in many European regions, traditional European medicine has a long and illustrious past in the treatment of a range of diseases **[34, 35].**

The pharmacological characteristics of therapeutic botanicals

Among these benefits are antidiabetic, anticancer, antimicrobial, immunomodulatory, antioxidant, antihyperlipidemic, antihypertensive, cardioprotective, and antiinflammatory effects, as well as protection from gastrointestinal diseases. The most often used herbal cures in conventional medicine for treating conditions like diabetes mellitus, cancer, infections, cardiovascular problems, inflammatory diseases, and gastrointestinal problems have been fully documented together with their respective pharmacological mechanisms **[36- 38].**

Type 2 Diabetes Mellitus (T2DM)

A range of metabolic diseases marked by extended elevated blood sugar levels brought on by problems affecting insulin production, release, or action, type 2 diabetes mellitus is Various herbal treatments including bioactive components from plants have been used throughout traditional medicine to treat type 2 diabetes and have proven to be effective in controlling blood glucose levels, restoring β-cell function, improving glucose tolerance and uptake, boosting insulin production and sensitivity, and lowering the development of reactive oxygen species connected to diabetes. **[39-41]**

Cancer

Multiple studies have indicated that herbal cures can suppress cancer cell development by reducing the activation of signaling chemicals such as NF-κB and TNF-α, therefore lowering tumor size, weight, load, and frequency. **[42-44].**

Infectious Diseases

In recent years, infectious diseases have become a prominent concern in the realm of global health. The medicinal properties of certain plants have been observed to exhibit antimicrobial or antiviral effects, curbing the proliferation of bacteria through interference with cell wall and protein synthesis, and preventing viral gene expression and invasion of host cells. Due to the escalation of drug-resistant microorganisms, there is an increasing focus on exploring the antimicrobial capacities of medicinal plants **[45- 50].**

Cardiovascular Diseases

Cardiovascular disease, which is the primary cause of death on a global scale, can be efficiently controlled by employing medicinal plants. Plant-based remedies with a long history in traditional medicine have been employed to treat cardiovascular diseases. The active components present in plant extracts have exhibited properties that protect the heart and lower blood pressure, in part due to actions like activating peroxisome proliferator-activated receptor γ (PPARγ) and blocking calcium influ. **[51- 53].**

Inflammatory Diseases

Adverse reactions may be reduced when medicinal herbs are used to treat inflammatory conditions. Through a number of processes, such as boosting antioxidant activity, inhibiting enzymes, and controlling gene expression, these herbs and their active ingredients have demonstrated anti-inflammatory qualities. They can also inhibit the production of prostaglandins and leukocyte adhesion. **[54].**

Gastrointestinal Disorders

Using a variety of strategies, phytotherapeutic treatments have proven effective in protecting the gastrointestinal tract from acid reflux. These include inhibiting H+/K+-ATPase activity, modifying GHR sensitivity to control cravings, increasing CCK and GLP-1 secretion, controlling fasting leptin levels, enhancing stomach motility, reducing abdominal pain associated with L-type calcium channels, inhibiting 5-HT3 receptors associated with symptoms of indigestion, controlling α2-adrenergic receptors, and monitoring mucus production. **[53].** Medicinal plants' biologically active substances and how they work as medicines ، known as phytochemicals, phytomolecules, or bio-nutrients, medicinal plants are rich in a wide variety of phytoconstituents. These molecules have a variety of structures. [**55- 59**].

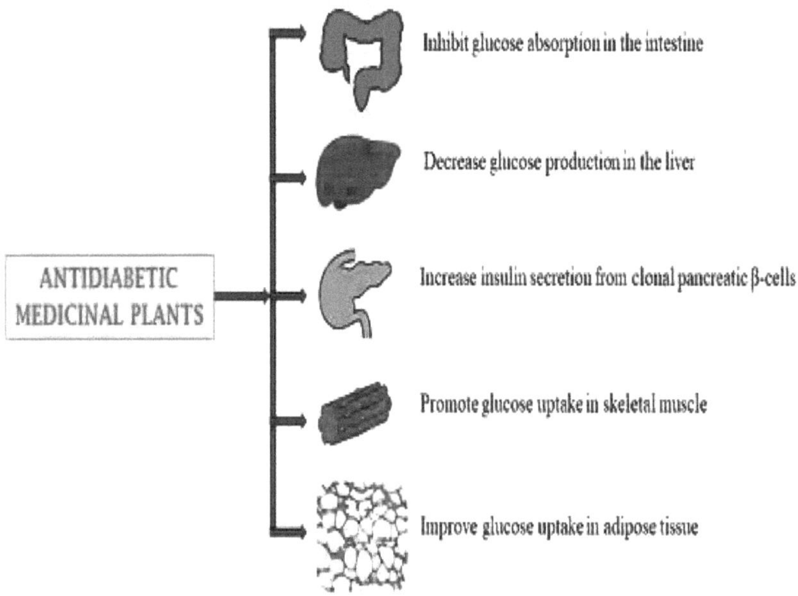

Figure 1. The particular organs and tissues impacted by medicinal plants used to treat diabetes are depicted in the schematic diagram.

Cancer

Cancer is a widespread disease that affects nations of all economic levels. The potential effectiveness of natural plant-based cancer treatments has drawn more attention since chemicals derived from plants, such as phytoconstituents and their derivatives, have showed promise as alternative medicines for cancer patients. **[60- 63]**

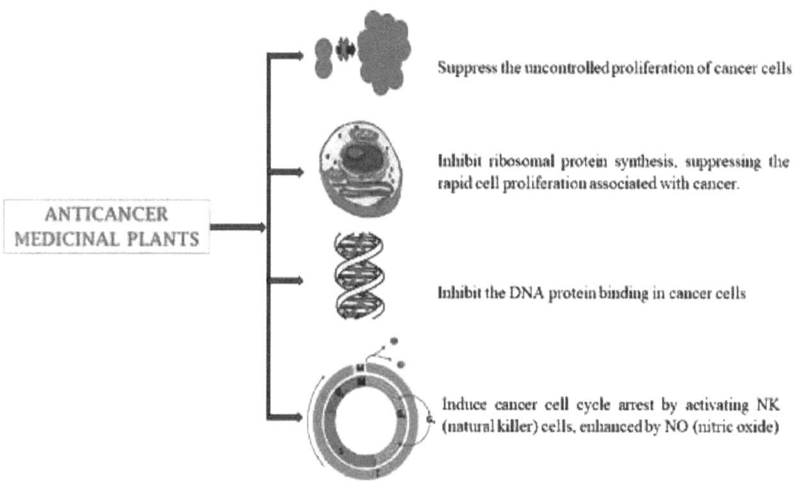

Figure 2. Illustration showing the specific organ or tissue targeted by medicinal plants used in anticancer treatment

Infectious Diseases

The rising global alarm regarding antimicrobial resistance (AMR) has prompted an increased emphasis on investigating alternative therapeutic options beyond traditional antibiotics.

Numerous plant compounds have displayed antimicrobial properties and have exhibited promising efficacy against multidrug-resistant strains of both Gram-negative and Gram-positive bacteria. Phytoconstituents such as allicin, spirostanol azadirone, nimbin, gedunin, euxanthone, harunmadagascarin D, piperine, reserpine, berberine, chelerythrine, allitridin, quercetin, dictamnine, ellagic acid, gallic acid, and aloe-emodin are among those that have demonstrated potential in this area [**64** - **68**].

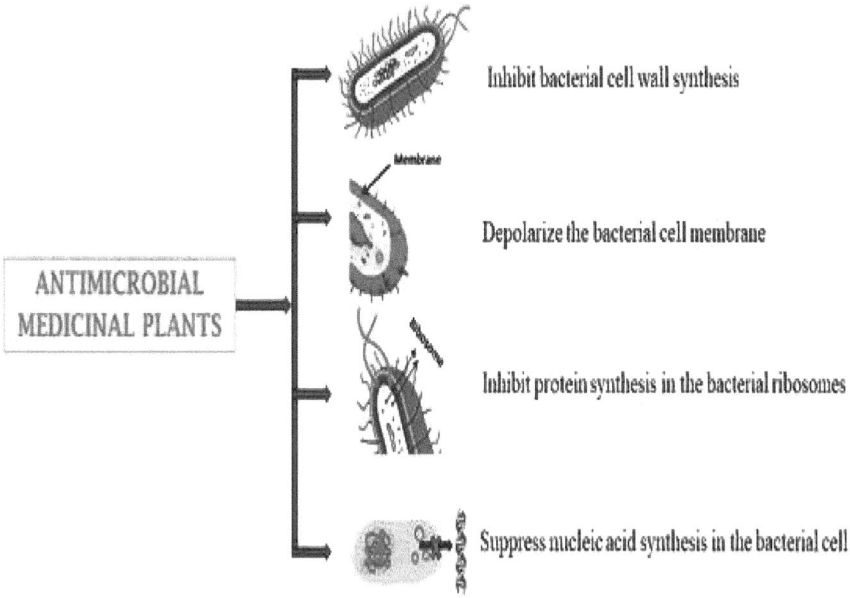

Figure 3. The schematic diagram depicts the specific organs and tissues that antimicrobial medicinal plants are intended to affect.

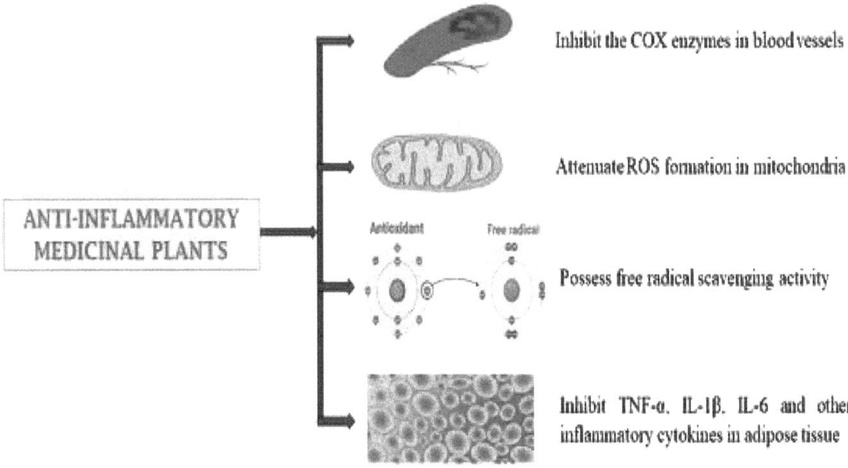

Figure 4. An illustrative diagram showing the precise organs and tissues affected by anti-inflammatory botanical remedies

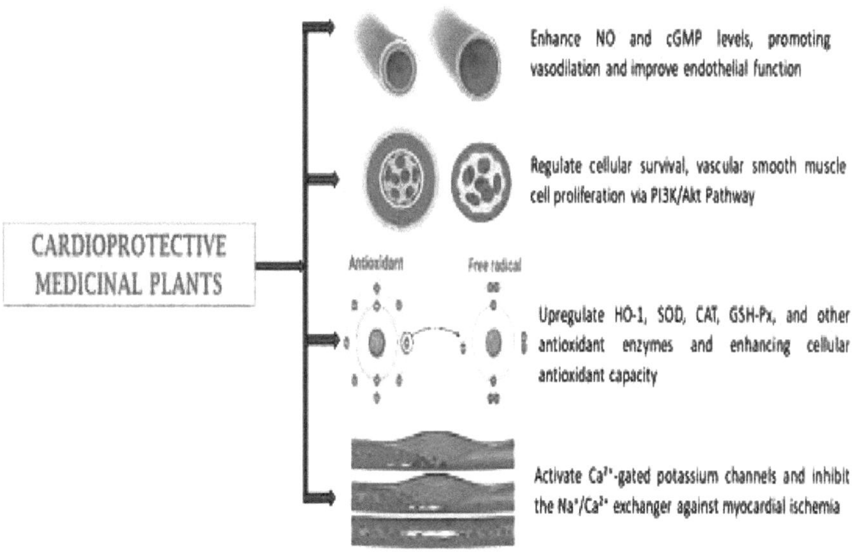

Figure 5. Illustrative diagram portraying the various mechanisms through which medicinal plants exhibit cardioprotective effects

Gastrointestinal Disorders

The global prevalence of gastrointestinal (GI) disorders is on the rise, attributed to the rapid process of globalization and shifts in lifestyle, particularly dietary patterns.

Quercitrin demonstrates the ability to regulate the metabolism of arachidonic acid, inhibit COX and lipoxygenase activity, lower the availability of Ca2+ during phases related to excitation-contraction coupling, reduce contractility in the ileum and jejunum, block 5-HT3 receptors, counteract the effects of 5-HT4 agonists, activate the PPARγ pathway, boost acetylcholine levels to facilitate gastric motility and emptying, increase motility in the stomach and proximal small bowel, and alleviate pain by inhibiting muscarinic receptors (Figure 6) [**69- 73**].

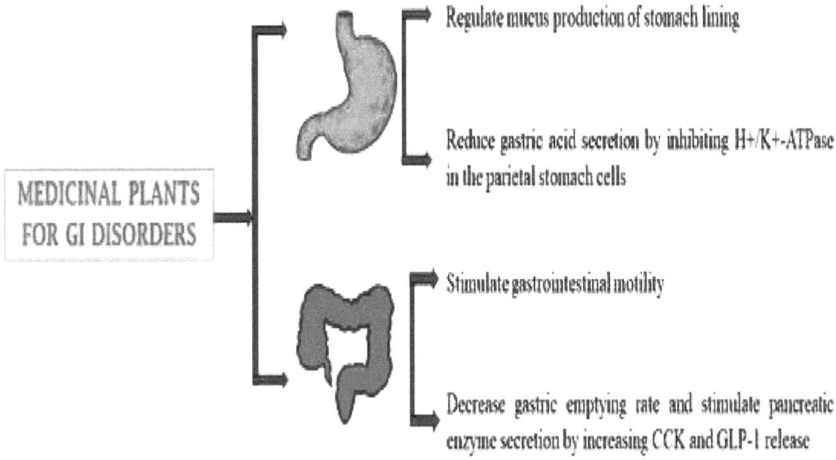

Figure 6. An example of the specific organs and tissues affected by medicinal plants used to treat ulcers shows how

Phytochemicals, for instance, enhance metabolic signaling and glucose absorption while inhibiting the enzymes that elevate blood sugar levels in the treatment of type 2 diabetes.

Additionally, phytochemicals have anti-inflammatory properties via reducing oxidative stress and cytokine activity as well as by targeting microbial proteins and enzymes to combat infections.

Considerable advantages to take into account include better availability, cost effectiveness, and fewer adverse reactions when compared to traditional medications. [**74-80**].

However, other phytochemicals, such as curcumin, have a limited rate of absorption and a slow onset of action, which prevents them from being widely used in medicine. Thus, increasing the bioavailability of plant-based medicines is a crucial subject for further study [**81- 83**].

For instance, quercetin is used to treat Type 2 Diabetes Mellitus and kaempferol have shown promising results in enhancing glycemic control by regulating the activities of α-glucosidase and GLUT4 [84, 85].

Because curcumin and quercetin can modulate PPARα, PI3K/Akt, and acetylcholinesterase, they have been identified as potential agents for the fight against cardiovascular diseases and can help maintain heart health.[**86**,87].

These novel techniques show, for example, how resveratrol activates Nrf2 to increase antioxidant protection against cardiovascular diseases, how curcumin inhibits NF-κB signaling to reduce the growth of cancer cells, and how epigallocatechin gallate inhibits COX-2 and IL-6 to reduce inflammation [**88**-93].

Ginger's phytochemical composition, therapeutic benefits, nutritional content and culinary uses

Numerous mechanisms, such as the body's inhibition of leukotrienes and prostaglandins to reduce inflammation, the activation of pain-relieving pathways, the interception of pain signals for analgesic effects, and the inhibition of cyclooxygenase-2 and tumor necrosis factor α in human synoviocytes, confirm ginger's therapeutic benefits.[**94**]

Despite the widespread belief that ginger is harmless, nothing is known about how its component parts function. Zingiber officinale Rosc, often known as ginger, is a perennial herbaceous plant that is indigenous to South-East Asia and belongs to the Zingiberaceae family. Numerous ailments, such as cancer, rheumatoid arthritis, and nausea, have been treated using gingerol, the primary component of ginger. [**95-100**].

There are many risk factors linked to human disease in the current day. These elements may be microbiological, such as viruses, bacteria, and fungi, or physical, such as exposure to heat, acid, cigarette smoke, and foreign objects. Knowing the different biological characteristics of popular plants, such as ginger, may help more people use their medical effects when needed. [**101**].

Botanical characteristics and geographic dispersion of the Ginger plant

The distribution of ginger was forecast to be worth US$7.03 billion in 2021. By 2029, total revenue is expected to have increased by 3.15%, to almost US$9.01 billion. The market has expanded as a result of the growing demand for ginger in the food and beverage industries **[102-104].**

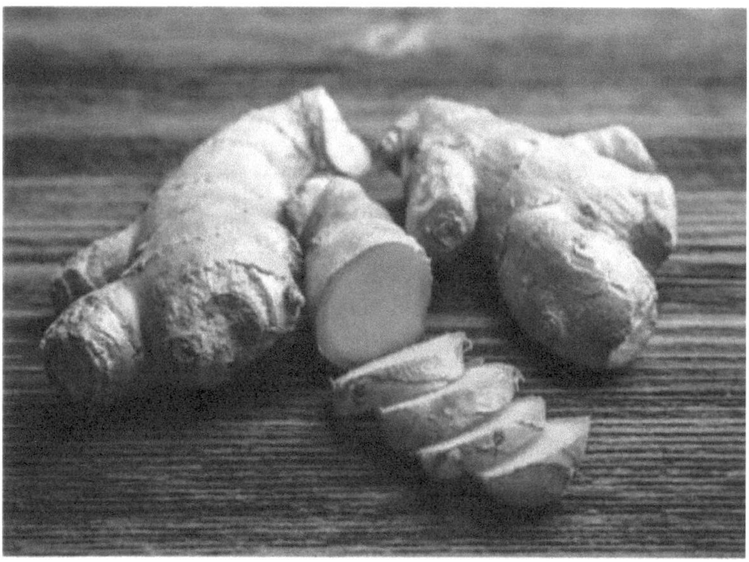

Fig. (7): Diagram of Ginger

Ginger nutrient content

Carbohydrate

The quantity of carbohydrates in each component used in meals should be taken into account by those who are regularly monitoring their carbohydrate consumption. Depending on their complexity and composition, carbohydrates can be divided into a number of classes. [**105- 107**].

Protein

The actual protein consumption from ginger alone is rather low because it is often used in small doses. Depending on factors including the type of ginger, how it is grown, and when it is harvested, the protein content of ginger might vary. [**108- 110**].

Inorganic nutrients

Ginger contains naturally occurring compounds called essential inorganic nutrients that give the body significant nutritional benefits. Ginger contains these essential inorganic elements that are required for regular bodily functions.

Phosphorus, a crucial inorganic ingredient for strong bones and teeth as well as energy metabolism, is also found in ginger **[111- 113].**

Bioactive compounds

Phenolic compounds

The conventional drying method of preservation may affect the phytochemical composition and antioxidant capability of ginger. Soluble phenolics found in ginger are markers of physiological changes caused by stress, which eventually because cell walls to stiffen. Additionally, by transforming phenolic compounds into flavonoids during the production of ginger, other beneficial plant products like anthocyanin, coumarin, and lignin can be created. It should be mentioned that the presence or absence of salicylic acid can affect ginger's photosynthetic rate under different light intensities. **[114- 117].**

Gingerol

According to studies, 6-gingerol has many pharmacological effects in addition to anti-inflammatory and antioxidant properties. **Fig. 8.**

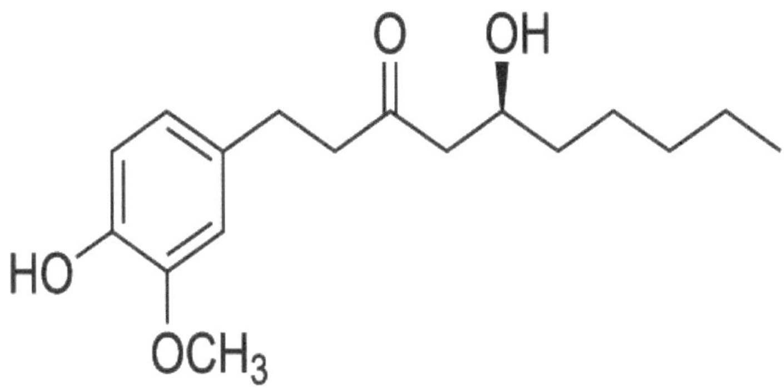

Fig. (8): The composition of gingerol in ginger

Shogaol

According to studies, this particular chemical has anti-inflammatory properties and can reduce inflammation by inhibiting the activity of lipoxygenase. Additionally, research has shown that 6-shogaol has antipyretic and analgesic qualities. [**118- 122**]. **Fig. 9**.

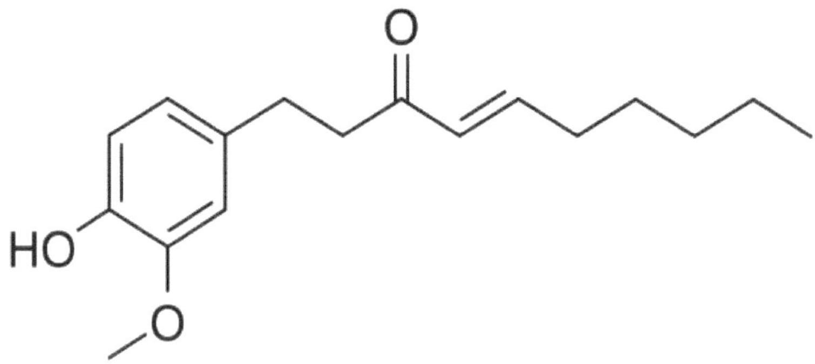

Fig. (9): Structure of shogaol

Paradols

Paradol's chemical structure has been defined, and its antioxidant and anticancer effects have been demonstrated through study using a mouse model. **Fig. 10.**

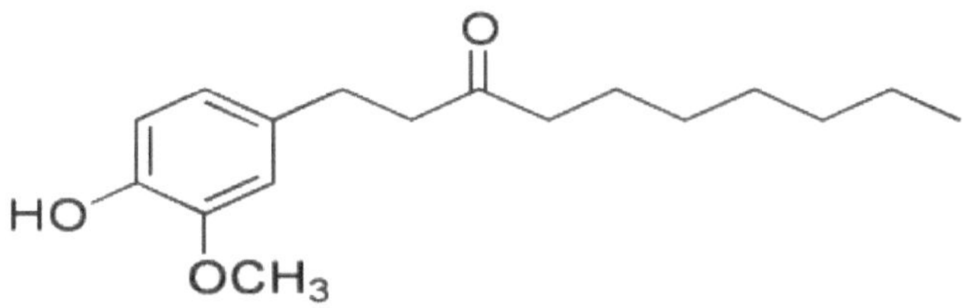

Fig. (10): Paradol's structure in ginger

Carotenoids

The amount of leaf carotenoids (LCC) is a crucial measure of the physiological health of the plant and is necessary for photosynthesis. When taken with lipids, carotenoids are more easily absorbed in the human diet. **[123- 126].**

Terpenoids

The key terpenoids in ginger are gingerol and geraniol, which represent the plant's numerous health benefits and also give it its distinctive smell. For example, these compounds possess different properties conferring antioxidant, and anti-inflammatory, antimicrobial and anticancer effects.

The concentration and composition of terpenoids in ginger can be influenced by the strain, growth conditions, and processing procedures employed, as it has to be taken into consideration. Therefore, the terpenoid profile of ginger and its therapeutic properties depend to a large extent on quality and bottling method of product. **[127- 131].**

Glycosides

These acetal derivatives produced by the interaction of an acid catalyst with a monosaccharide or alcohol Ginger's stored chemicals are passive glycosides that enzymes can hydrolyze to become active. **[132- 134]**

This method makes the sugar component accessible by removing the active chemical moiety. Medicine has discovered advantages of ginger glycosides. The word "alkaloids" is nearly improper as glycosides lack nitrogen. For ginger, glycosides serve several critical purposes. **[135- 138]**

Tannins

Tannin molecules present in ginger plants act as natural insecticides, protecting the plant from predators and perhaps controlling growth.

Moreover, tannins in the bark of ginger plants help to avoid fungal and bacterial infections. Changes in tannin composition across time will have a big influence on the ideal times to harvest plants high in proanthocyanidins, a type of tannin having molecular weights ranging from 500 to more than 20,000 Daltons. **[139- 143]**.

Oxalates

The elevated levels of typically soluble sodium urate, a crucial component of gout, seem to be significantly influenced by the presence of very insoluble iron (II) oxalate. There has been a lot of research on oxalate metabolism in animals, fungi, and ginger, but little is known about it in plants. The biomineral oxalate, which is present in many tissues and organs, is commonly found in ginger in a variety of crystalline forms. It is frequently found in the vacuoles of tiger nut specialized cells known as crystal idioblasts. **[144- 151].**

Biological activities of ginger

Antioxidant properties

The main cause of chemotherapy-induced nausea and vomiting (CINV) is the production of toxic free radicals in the digestive tract, which sets off the release of neurotransmitters by enterochromaffin cells that result in vomiting. **[152- 160].**

Antifertility properties

Research has been conducted to investigate the possible health benefits of ginger. However, little is known about its antifertility qualities. Most studies on the effects of ginger on fertility are based on laboratory or animal investigations. Ginger is frequently recommended and used to help expecting mothers who are experiencing motion sickness. **[160- 163]**

Ginger's potential to reduce nausea brought on by gynecological laparoscopy has been the subject of several research **[164, 165]. Fig.11**

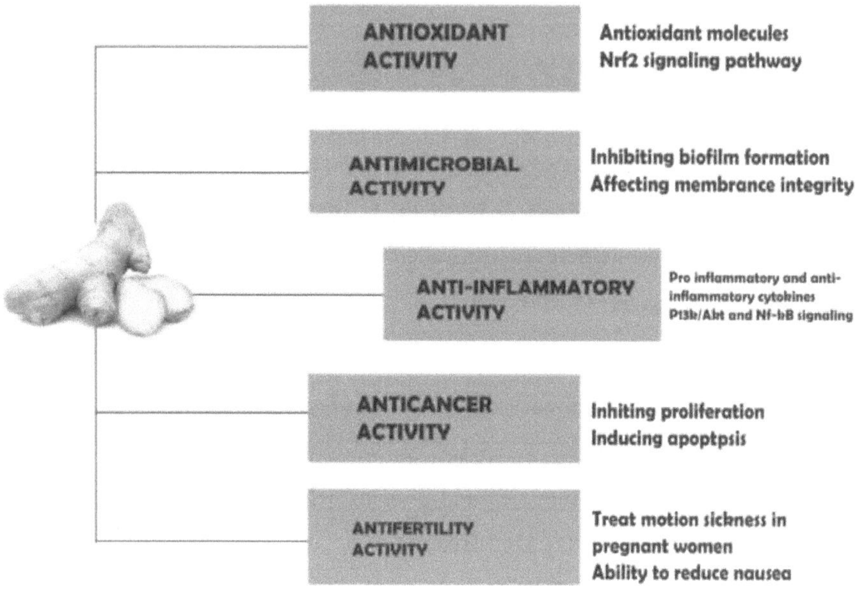

Fig. (11): Ginger's biological actions

Antisickling potential

Recent research reveals that ginger may have properties that would stop red blood cells from sickling, a common indication of sickle cell disease. Preliminary studies indicate that some chemicals present in ginger might inhibit the production of red blood cells with anomalous shapes. **[166–168]**

Recent studies indicate that ginger and other herbal remedies might have anti-sickling effects, therefore offering a new treatment option for persons suffering from this hemoglobin condition. **[169- 171].Fig. 12**

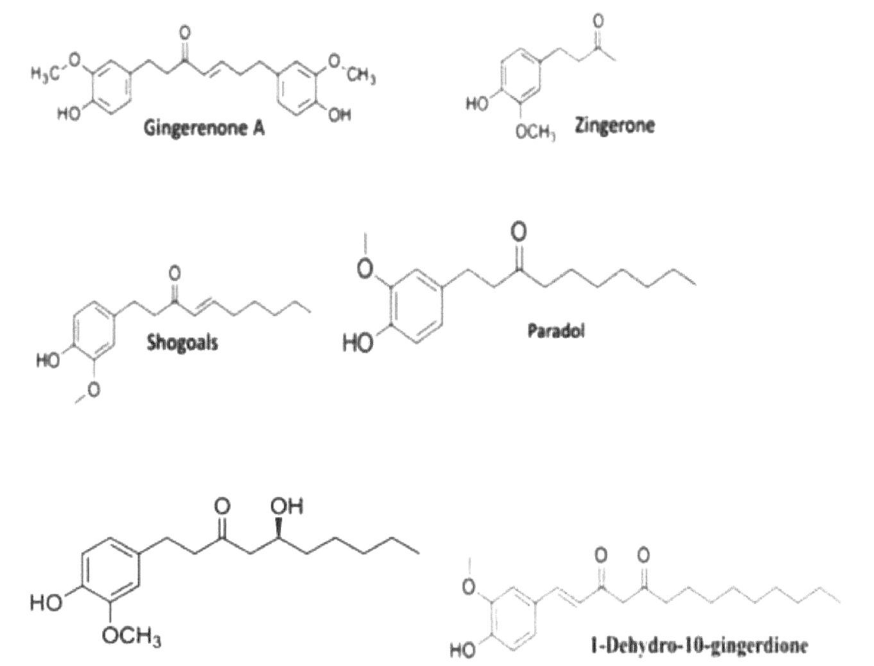

Fig. (12): The molecular makeup of the key ingredient in ginger that helps prevent sickle cell anemia.

Anti-obesity properties

An increased risk of acquiring a number of chronic diseases, including diabetes, hypertension, and cardiovascular disorders, has been linked to obesity. Ginger may provide benefits in treating and preventing obesity, according to several studies. Specifically, compared to gingerols and 6-shogaol, gingerenone A has been demonstrated to have a more marked ability to suppress the creation of fat cells and the accumulation of lipids in early fat cells. Gingerenone A's stimulation of AMPK in living things may help control the metabolism of fat and lessen diet-induced obesity. **[171- 176]. Fig. 13**

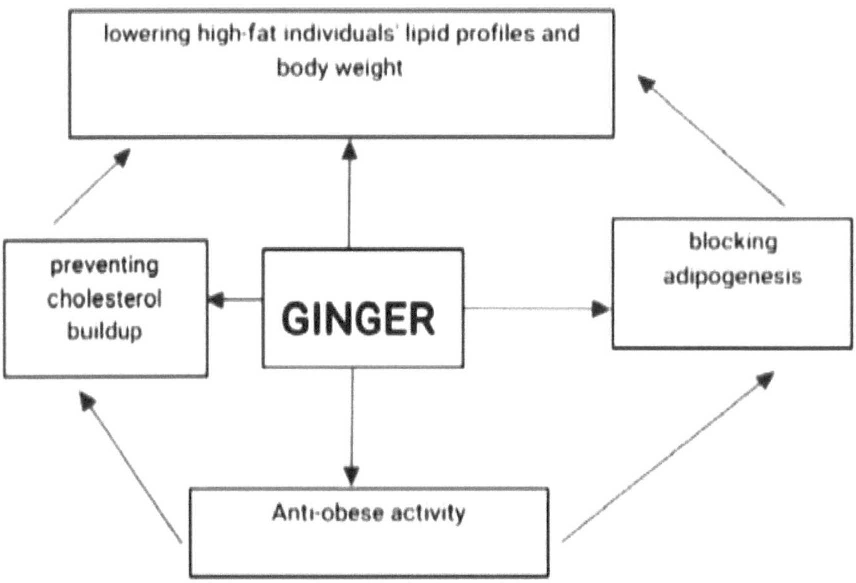

Fig. (13): Ginger and its components play a significant role in the management of obesity

Anti diabetic property

A research study examining the effects of ginger on diabetes revealed that the compound 6-gingerol can increase insulin secretion in response to glucose and improve glucose tolerance in type 2 diabetic mice by enhancing levels of glucagon-like peptide 1. Additionally, it was shown that this substance increases the expression of glucose transporter type 4 on cell membranes and activates glycogen synthase 1, which increases the amount of glycogen stored in skeletal muscles. Ginger use has also been demonstrated to lower triglycerides and fasting plasma glucose levels in diabetics.

In conclusion, the potential of ginger and its derivatives to offer protection against diabetes and its related problems has been demonstrated by a number of investigations and clinical trials. **[177- 179].Fig. 14**

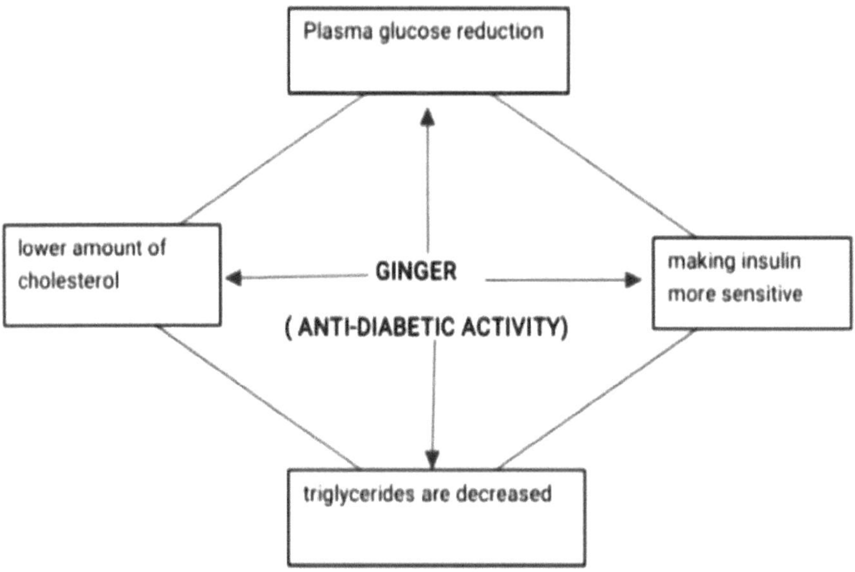

Fig. (14): Recent studies have shown that ginger and its constituents are effective in treating diabetes.

Ginger's hepatoprotective properties

Empirical evidence from earlier research has demonstrated that ginger and its constituents are important liver protectors. A significant study on ginger showed that it could shield the liver from toxicity caused by mancozeb and CCl_4. Certain minerals and chemical substances found in ginger contribute to its hepatoprotective qualities. **[180].**

Given these characteristics, ginger could be a rather successful all-natural treatment for stomach ulcers. Speaking with medical specialists is essential for an accurate diagnosis and suggestions on how to use ginger to treat certain medical conditions. **[181-183]. Fig. 15**

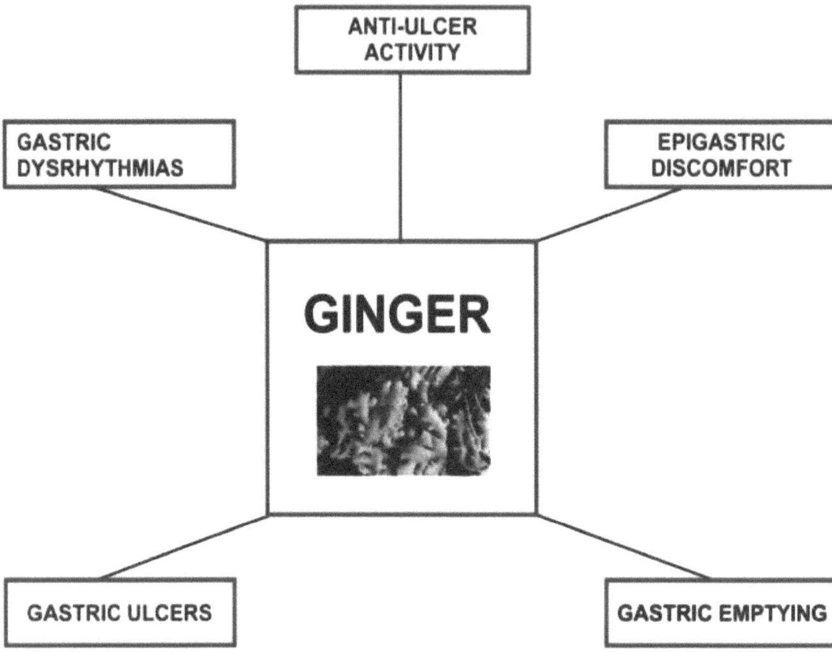

Fig. (15): It has been discovered that ginger offers qualities that could aid in the prevention and treatment of ulcers.

Ginger's industrial uses

Ginger is utilized in several industries, such as food, cosmetics, pharmaceuticals, and more, as seen in **Fig. 16. [184- 186]**

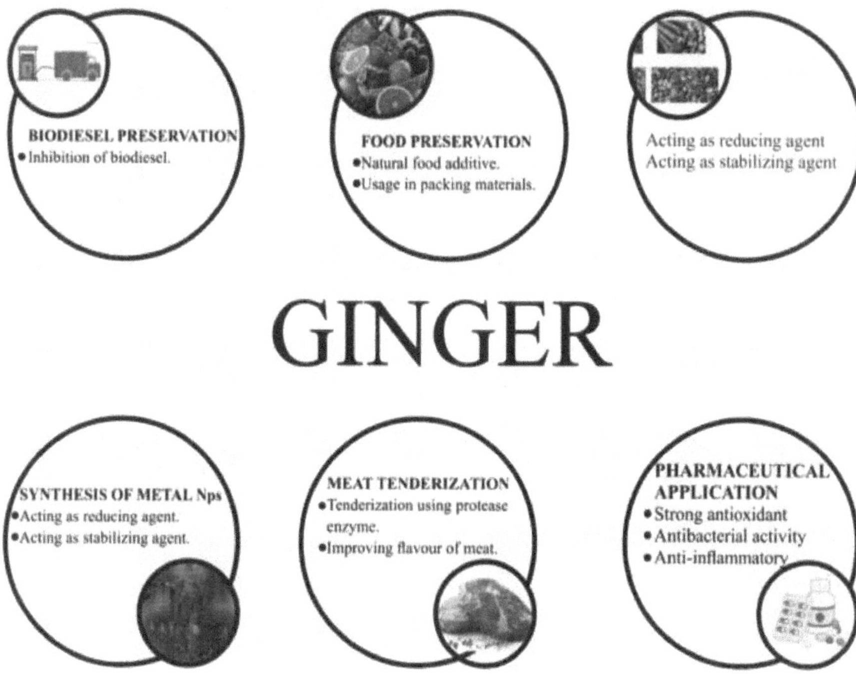

BIODIESEL PRESERVATION
• Inhibition of biodiesel.
FOOD PRESERVATION
• Natural food additive.
• Usage in packing materials.
Acting as reducing agent
Acting as stabilizing agent
GINGER
SYNTHESIS OF METAL Nps
• Acting as reducing agent.
• Acting as stabilizing agent.
MEAT TENDERIZATION
• Tenderization using protease enzyme.
• Improving flavour of meat.
PHARMACEUTICAL APPLICATION
• Strong antioxidant
• Antibacterial activity
• Anti-inflammatory

Fig. (16): Ginger's industrial uses

Garlic's efficacy, safety, and possible drawbacks

Research indicates that ginger extracts may be able to boost the synthesis of a number of harmful substances, including AF2 and NTG. A study found that the active component of gingerol is the hydroxyl group in the aliphatic chain moiety; shogaol, a component of ginger, may be less mutagenic than gingerol. **[187- 197].**

Polyphenols

Polyphenols have been discovered to offer a variety of health benefits, such as decreasing the negative effects of free radicals, providing protection against cardiovascular diseases, cancer, and age-related ailments. Furthermore, they have been shown to reduce inflammation and allergic responses.

In addition, flavonoids have demonstrated efficacy in treating a variety of conditions including angina pectoris, cervical lesions, chronic venous insufficiency, dermatopathy, diabetes, gastrointestinal disorders, lymphocytic leukemia, menopausal symptoms, rhinitis, traumatic cerebral infarction, among others. **[198-205].**

Phytosterols

Phytosterols refer to plant sterols and stanols that play a role in regulating various physiological functions in plants. **[206- 210]**

Campesterol is a sterol that is recognized for its straightforward structure, with the exception of the double bonds in the B-ring. It contains a hydroxyl group at position C-3 of the steroid skeleton, fully saturated bonds within its molecular framework, and a methyl group at C24. In contrast to campesterol, sitosterol, a variant of phytosterol, features a beta-hydroxy group at position 3 instead of the stigmast-5-ene moiety. **[211-215]**

Campestanol is categorized as a 3-beta-sterol, originating from 5-alpha-campestane. Stigmastanol belongs to the steroid family and has saturated bonds in the fifth and sixth places of the B-ring in addition to a hydroxyl group in the C-3 position of its steroid structure. This specific substance is a 3-hydroxy steroid that is produced from a 5-alpha-stigmastane hydride **[216, 217].**

Saponins

Another naturally occurring triterpenoid molecule, oleanane, is a member of the oleanoid group and has six-membered rings that contain taxerol and beta-amyrin. The tetracyclic triterpenoid saponin tirucallane, which is mostly found in euphorbia, has several advantageous qualities, including hypoglycemia, virucidal, antifungal, antibacterial, and hypolipidemic actions **[218- 222].**

Polysaccharides and Dietary Fibers

These substances serve as either indigestible substances or molecules that store energy, such as glycogen and starch. Consuming dietary fiber regularly can prevent a number of health problems, including cancer, inflammation, hypertension, hyperlipidemia, hypercholesterolemia, obesity, and cardiovascular diseases **[223- 227].**

Phytochemical Extraction Methods

The process of removing or acquiring desirable chemicals from source material is referred to as extraction. Because of its non-selective qualities, which enable the separation of hydrophilic materials like saponins, phenolics, and polysaccharides, water in particular is acknowledged as the most popular and adaptable solvent **[228- 232].**

Maceration

The efficiency of the extraction process depends on a number of variables, including the solvent selection, extraction time, temperature, and food matrix composition. Maximum extraction is possible with this technique while using the least amount of solvent. The efficiency of the extraction process is explained in depth in relation to the polarity of the solvents utilized. Thermolabile chemicals are preserved through extraction processes that are carried out at lower temperatures without the use of heat. **[233- 235] Fig. 17.**

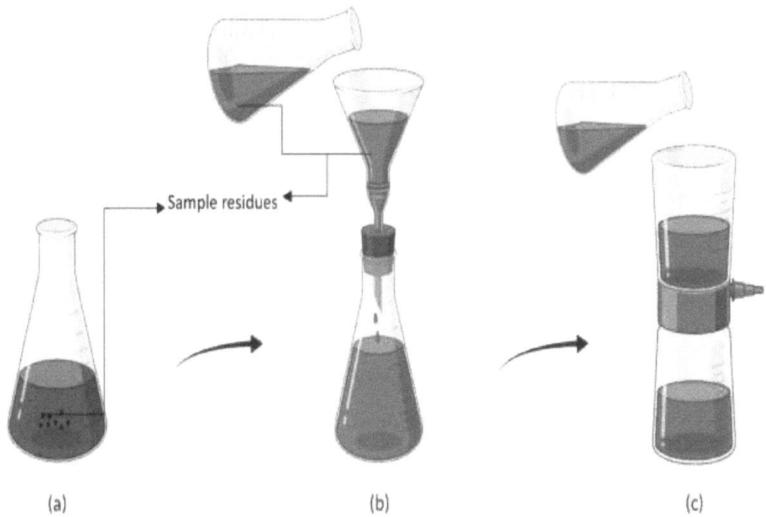

Fig. (17) A number of crucial processes are involved in maceration extraction. First, the material is mixed with a solvent and allowed to sit for seven days.

Percolation

As shown in Figure 18, this complex procedure starts with submerging the plant sample in a large volume of solvent before moving it to a sealed container for a predetermined duration of time. In order to guarantee consistent liquid distribution and flow, the sample must be carefully introduced into the percolator before it is filled and sealed. A steady percolation rate, which indicates the best way for the sample to pass through the various levels of the percolator, depends on the bottom outlet's controlled release. After that, more solvent is added to completely saturate the material in the percolator for a predetermined amount of time. 24 hours. Repercolation, which involves repeatedly passing the solvent and sample through a network of interconnected percolators, is a major breakthrough in the percolation technique **[234- 240]. Fig. 18**

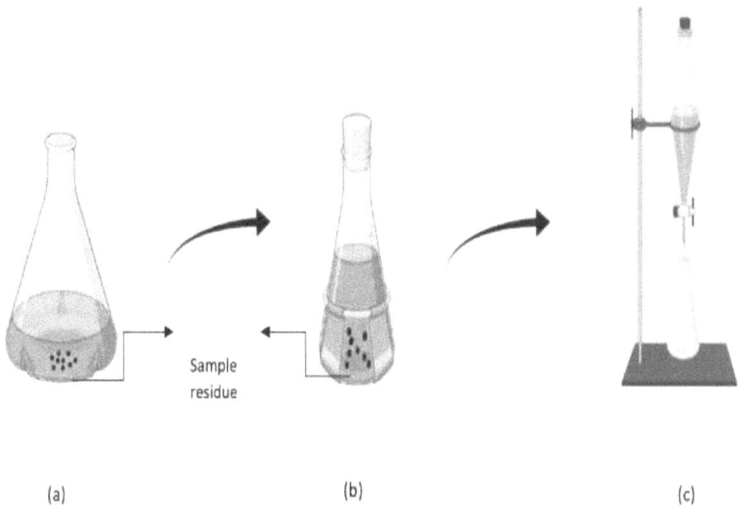

Fig. (18) A graphic representation of the percolation extraction procedure is shown. The sample is first immersed in a solvent. The sample is then moved to a sealed decanter and given four hours to sit. Using a percolator to filter out the materials completes the extraction process.

Decoction

The plant material is strained through multiple layers of muslin cloth after being boiled in water for a specific period of time. Other techniques, such centrifugation and the solvent evaporating from the supernatant, can be employed to improve extraction. Extraction is often carried out at a fixed temperature for a set period of time in order to get the optimum results. By inhibiting glucuronidase activity during the decoction process with high temperatures, glycosides are preserved and the final extract contains more flavones **[241]. Fig. 19**

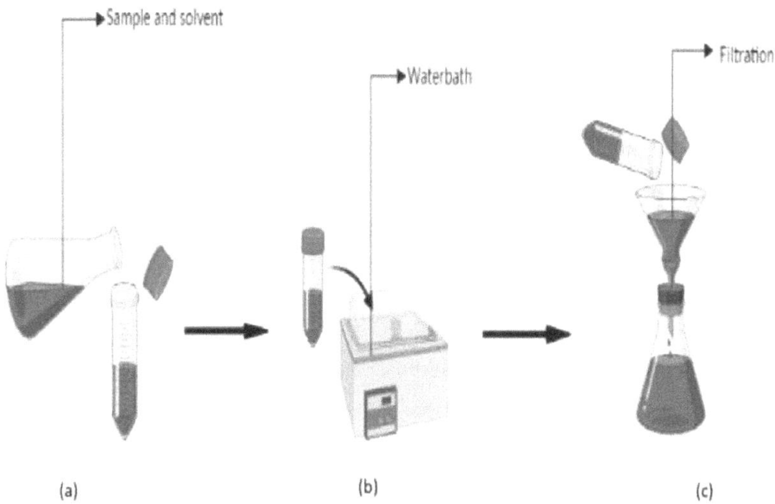

Fig. (19) The following figure shows the decoction extraction process: (a) The sample is put in a sealed glass tube, and (b) it is submerged for 30 to 2 hours at a temperature of 65 to 70 °C in a water bath. (c) The extract is filtered after this procedure.

Reflux Extraction

The solid-liquid extraction process used in the reflux extraction method, as shown in Figure 22, involves solvent evaporation and condensation for one to three hours at a constant temperature range of 60 to 80°C. This approach is widely used. Temperatures between 60 and 80°C and extraction times between 80 and 120 minutes are typical extraction conditions using a mixture of solvents like ethanol and water. The boiling point of the solvent and the length of the extraction process are the main determining factors, and the extraction efficiency using this method usually ranges from 70 to 90%. Depending on the particular criteria being followed, the extraction period should be extended till it reaches asymptotic levels or exhaustive phases **[241, 242]. Fig. 20**

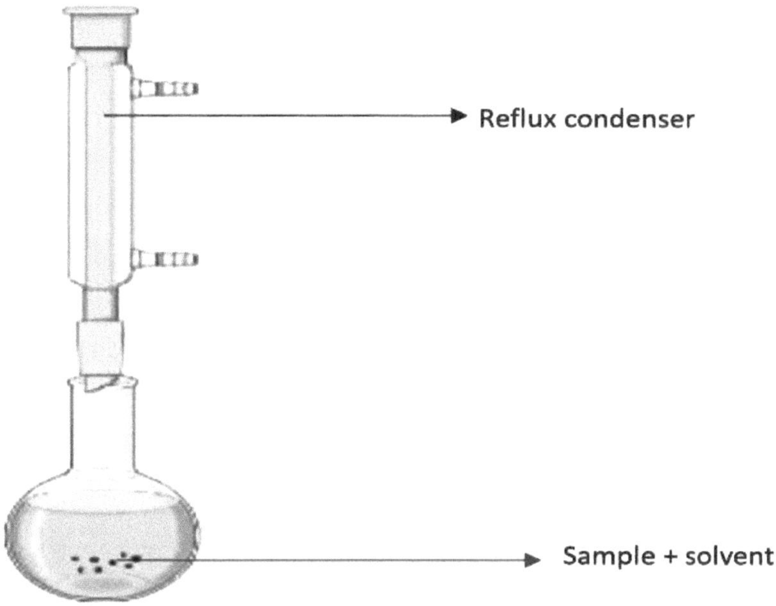

Fig. (20) An example of the reflux extraction procedure

Soxhlet Extraction

Using the Soxhlet extraction method, a little amount of dried material is placed in a thimble and then placed in a distillation flask that is filled with various solvents, such as hexane, toluene, and petroleum ether (see Fig. 23). This technique is well known for its effectiveness and continuous extraction process, which requires less time and solvent than maceration or percolation. **[243- 246].**

Because of the possibility of flavonoid degradation, samples with a high water content are not appropriate for extraction using this method. There are further environmental issues with disposing of the used solvent. High extraction temperatures may also cause the target chemical to thermally decompose. **[247].**

Fig. 21.

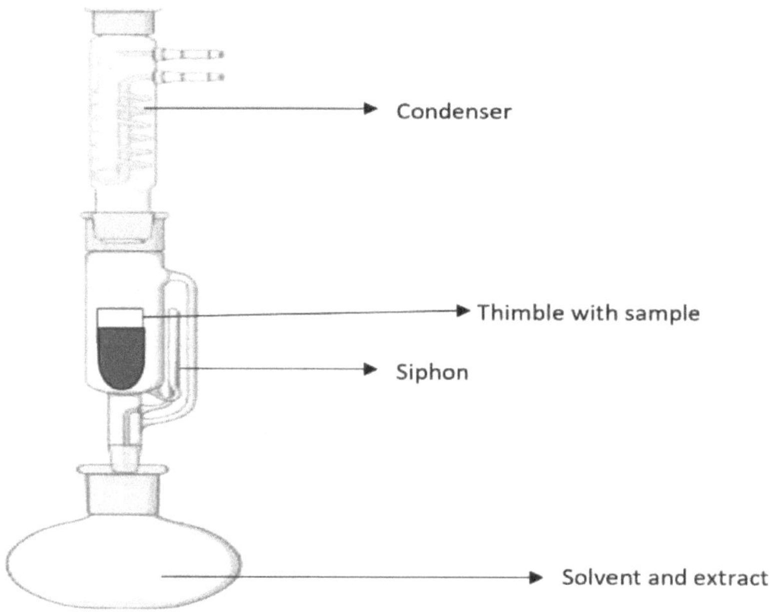

Fig. (21) An illustration of the Soxhlet extraction procedure.

Pressurized Liquid Extraction

Analytes can be effectively extracted from a solid matrix using pressurized liquid extraction (PLE), which uses liquid solvents, high temperature, and pressure. This technique is unique in that it has broad solubility and mass transfer qualities. PLE functions in the range of 50 to 200 °C and 50 to 300 psi of pressure. Compared to Soxhlet extraction, PLE takes less time and uses less solvents. This method, which uses organic solvents in place of CO_2, is often seen as a natural replacement for supercritical fluid extraction. Because PLE uses less solvents, it is also considered a sustainable or eco-friendly extraction technique. Large extract dilutions, poor analyte selectivity, potential interfering chemicals, and the need for complex equipment are the main obstacles to the widespread use of PLE **[248- 252]. Fig. 22.**

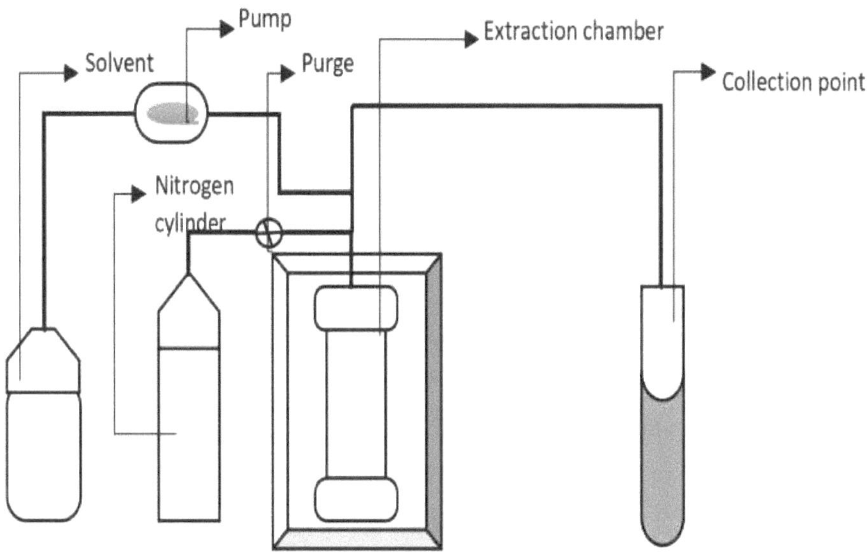

Fig. (22) An illustration of a liquid extraction process under pressure.

Liquid Gas Extraction

Both isobaric and non-isobaric techniques can be used in the extraction process; isobaric extraction uses continuous pressure to move the solvent without the need for a compressor or pump, while non-isobaric extraction uses a pump to transfer liquefied gas through the raw material. Lipids, carotenoids, terpenoids, and other substances can be extracted using liquid gas extraction technology.

Research indicates that using liquefied petroleum gas may lessen the breakdown or modification of phytochemicals. However, a major disadvantage of this strategy is its high cost, which results from the requirement for specialized storage facilities and transportation vehicles due to the high pressure and low temperature required to keep and transport the solvent in liquid form. Lipids, carotenoids, terpenoids, and other substances can be extracted using liquid gas extraction technology.

Research indicates that using liquefied petroleum gas may lessen the breakdown or modification of phytochemicals. However, a major disadvantage of this strategy is its high cost, which results from the requirement for specialized storage facilities and transportation vehicles due to the high pressure and low temperature required to keep and transport the solvent in liquid form. Lipids, carotenoids, terpenoids, and other substances can be extracted using liquid gas extraction technique; studies show that using liquefied petroleum gas reduces the breakdown or modification of phytochemicals.

However, a major drawback of this strategy is its high cost, which is related to the requirement for specialized storage facilities and transportation vehicles due to the high pressure and low temperature required to store and transport the solvent in its liquid condition **[253, 254].**

Microwave-Assisted Extraction

The usual frequencies at which microwave devices function are 915 MHz and 2450 MHz. Significant ablation zones with a significant depth of electromagnetic energy penetration are created when microwaves operating at 915 MHz are used. Conversely, dipoles align and randomize about 4.9 × 109 at 2450 MHz. times per second, leading to molecular movement through friction and subsequent solution heating **[253- 258]. Fig. 23.**

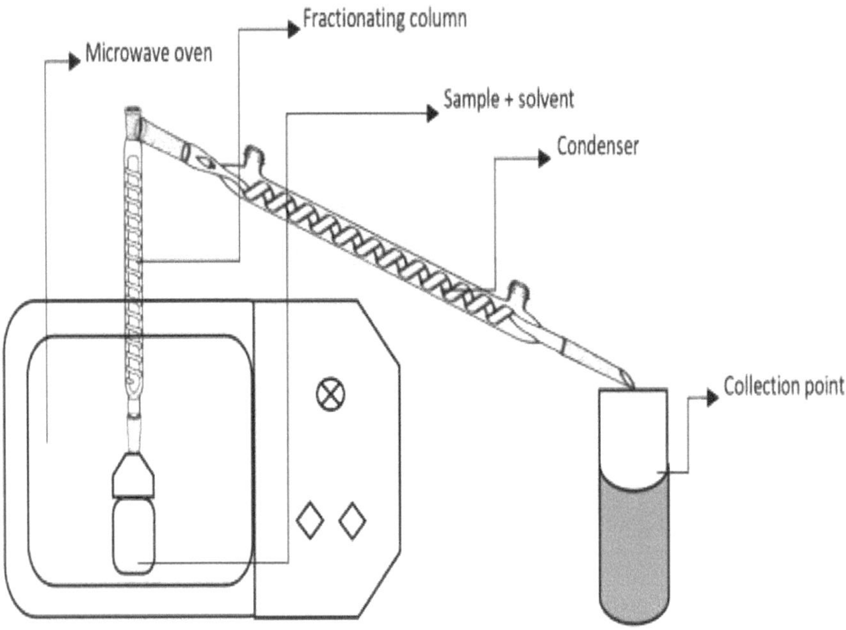

Fig. (23) A graphic representation of the microwave-enhanced extraction procedure

Ultrasound-Assisted Extraction

A technique that takes advantage of the phenomenon of acoustic or ultrasonic cavitation is called ultrasonic extraction, or ultrasound-assisted extraction (UAE). A probe-type ultrasonic processor creates acoustic coupling in a slurry using high-power ultrasonic pulses, starting cycles of high and low pressure to flow through the liquid (Figure 24).

The effectiveness of ultrasonic-assisted extraction (UAE) is significantly influenced by a number of variables, including the kind of solvent and its characteristics, the length of extraction, temperature, power levels, and the presence of gases.

The widespread application of UAE for the extraction of phytochemicals from complicated matrices, such algae, is hindered by challenges in accurately regulating power levels, which leads to inefficient energy transmission within the extraction vessel **[258-260]. Fig. 24.**

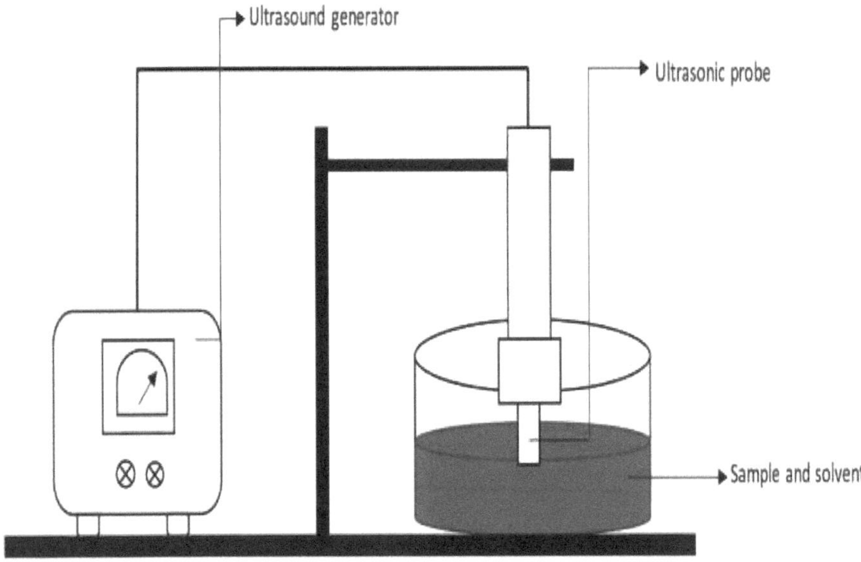

Fig. (24) An illustration of extraction with ultrasound assistance.

Pulsed Electric Field Extraction

By increasing the sample's cell membranes' conductivity, porosity, and permeability, this technique makes it easier for materials contained within the membrane to move into the surrounding fluid **[561- 564]. Fig. 25.**

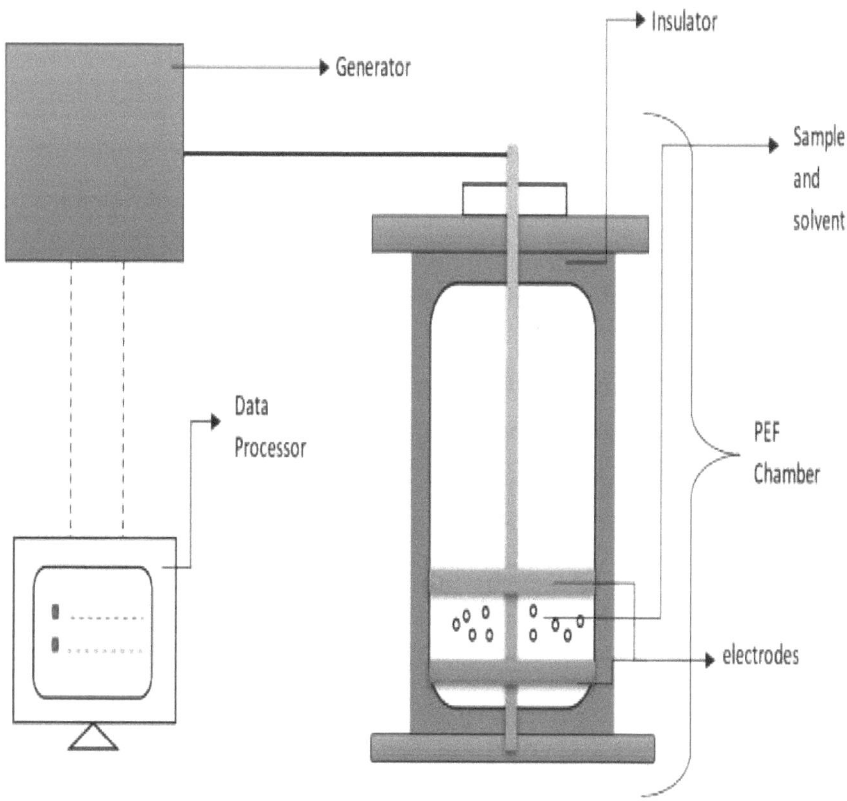

Fig. (25): An example of the removal of materials using pulsed electric fields.

Enzyme Assisted Extraction

Enzymes are used as powerful catalysts in order to isolate, transform and make synthetic complex bioactive molecules using the natural sources. Their outstanding ability to speed up responses (Fig. 28) offers one of the alternatives to the traditional solvent-based technologies and increases sustainability. The cellulases, hemicellulases, and pectinases are some of the most commonly used enzymes in the extraction of bioactive materials. These enzymes work through breaking plant cell walls and decreasing their structure.

Enzyme-assisted extraction is used to extract the oils that have a yield of about 38 -52 percent, a process usually carried out at 33 -67 o C and a time span of between 20-220 minutes. The activity and hydrolytic properties of the extraction process depend on numerous factors, among them being the sample composition, enzyme activity, constituent types in it, and enzyme concentrations. Further, temperature has a considerable impact on enzyme activity, where high temperatures make the medium extracting less viscous, which increases bioactive substance solubility.

To enhance catalytic efficiency, it is necessary to retain the acidic pH of 4.5 in order to alter the structures of proteins and expand substrate binding capacity. The prices of enzymes are very expensive and as such, they cannot be adopted on a large scale in extraction processes, they can only be applied on a few samples. There is still a problem of ensuring the total hydrolysis of plant cell walls to obtain highest possible phytochemical extraction yield, despite enzyme combinations progress **[265- 268]. Fig. 26.**

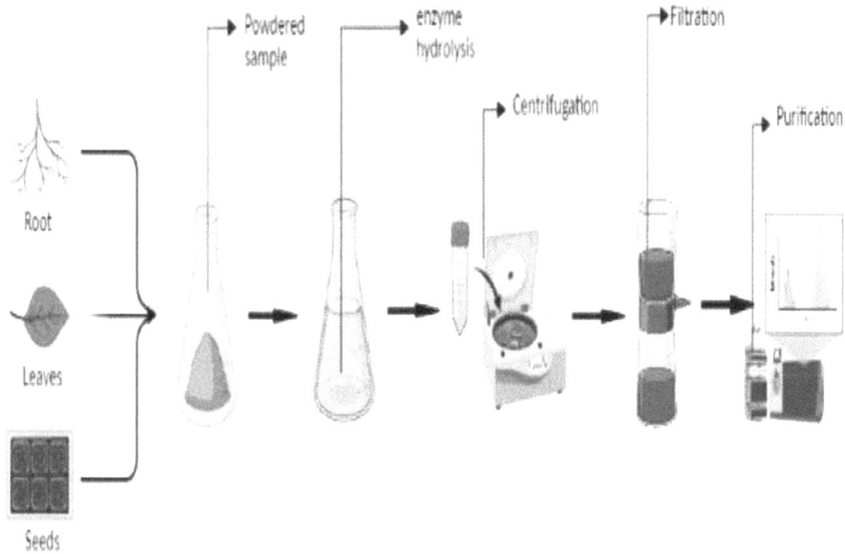

Fig. (26): An illustrative depiction of extraction facilitated by enzymes

Supercritical Fluid Extraction

The properties of a strong solvent and a high level of diffusivity are what makes supercritical CO 2 (SC-CO_2) highly attractive. It is notable that CO_2 is found in a gaseous state at the ambient temperature and pressure, hence producing extract without any solvent residue.

The extraction variables which have significant influence on the efficiency of the extraction process include extraction pressure, temperature, duration, solvent-to-material ratio as well as solvent flow rate **[269- 275]. Fig. 27.**

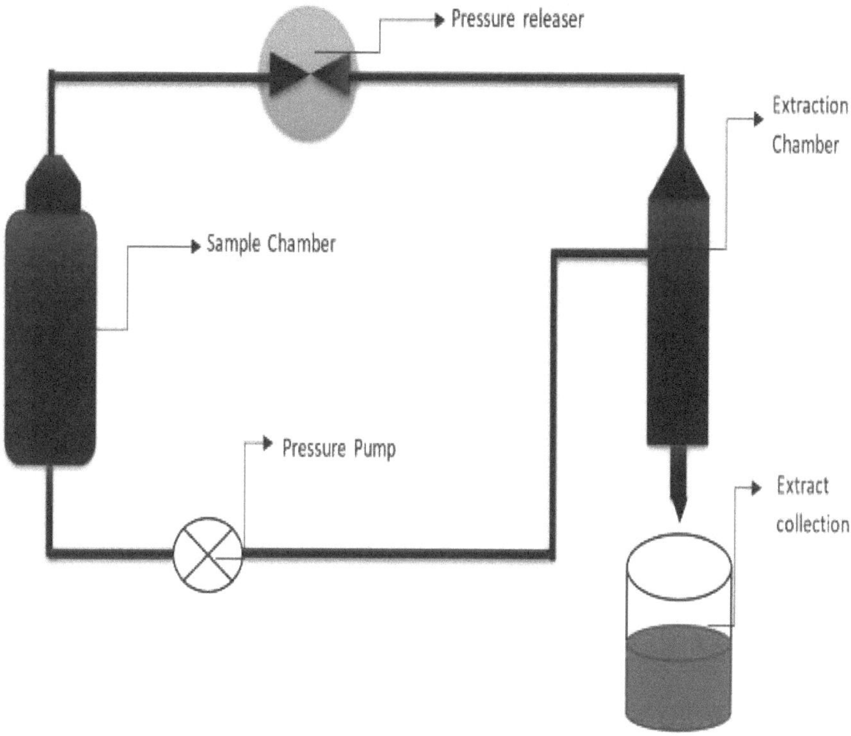

Fig. (27): An example of how supercritical fluid extraction works.

High Hydrostatic Pressure Processing

High hydrostatic pressure processing (HPP), which is a non-thermal intervention, commonly used to process liquid food, attempts to destroy microorganisms that cause disease and those that cause food spoilage by exposing the food to pressure between 400 and 600 Mega Pascal (MPa).

The pressure can sometimes be up to 1000 MPa. Unlike most of the traditional methods, HPP can be done at low temperature, mostly lower than 45 C and hence maintains the sensory properties and nutritional values of the food product. A sample of food is put into a vessel that is subjected to high hydrostatic pressure and mixed with a suitable solvent most commonly water used in industrial processes to extract HPP.

Alternative solvents can also be used in some areas of science, like ethanol, glycerol, silicon oil or solvent mixtures.

High pressure in HPP disrupts the cell walls releasing cytoplasm that contains bioactive compounds, which are then retrieved in the solvent. Since the level of pressure increases the solubility of soluble components, the effectiveness of this extraction technique highly depends on the amount of pressure used. The principle of the high hydrostatic pressure processing is thus explained in Fig.28. **[276-278].**

Fig. 28.

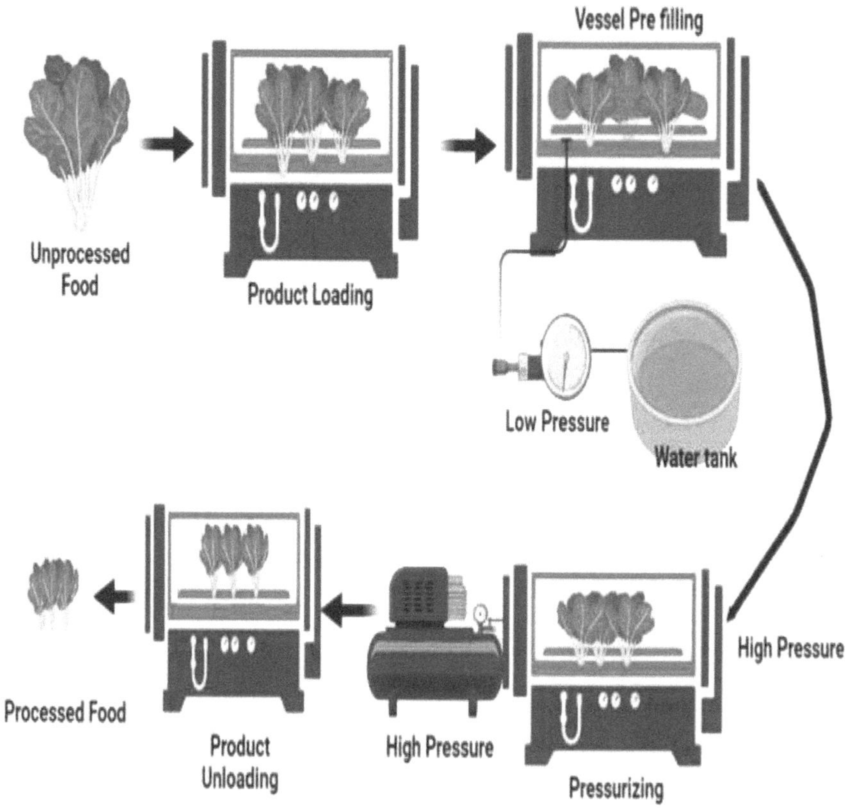

Fig. (28) :A schematic representation of the high hydrostatic pressure treatment method

Natural Deep Eutectic Solvent Extraction

NADES can be chemically modified to offer a change in their physical and chemical characteristics through a modification in their composition. Temperature and water content are considered to be important variables that affect the characteristics of NADES. The density and viscosity of NADES are lower with the addition of water, and the polarity is higher. Conductivity of the solvent and solubility of the solutes in NADES have a significant influence on water.

NADES have no specific melting point and have decomposition temperatures greater than 135 o C and glass transition temperatures less than 50 o C. As a result, NADES are used with solvents between the temperature of 0 and 100 o C. The extraction efficiency was found to be 62 0 -70 percent over the temperature range of 25 -105 0 C and 30-60 minutes of extraction time; the stability of the solvent mixture is strongly dependent on the extraction efficiency.

Chloroform is the most effective and popular hydrogen bond acceptor of dietary fibers and polysaccharides especially lignin. Curcumin is more soluble in a mannose-dimethylurea-water mixture of 2:5:5. The requirement of various ingredients into the making of eutectic solvents as well as the high viscosity that might compromise the stability are two significant drawbacks of Natural Deep Eutectic Solvents (NADES).

This makes NADES unsuitable for long-term storage since they are not as stable as other solvents and may, in fact, solidify. NADES should be prepared during extraction and are not advised to hold on to long **[279- 285]. Fig. 29.**

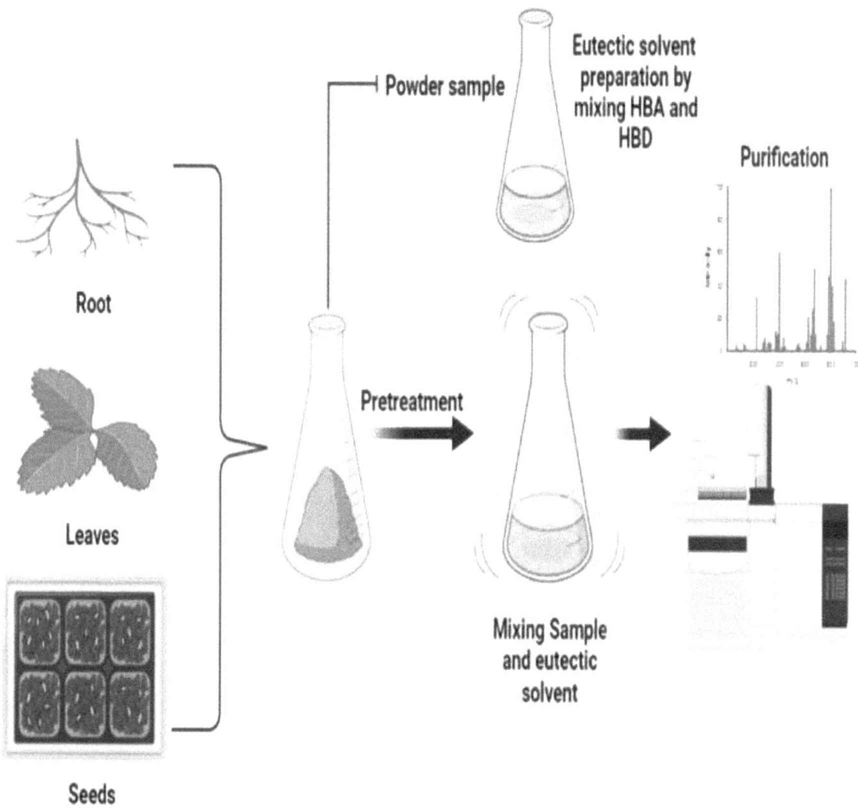

Fig. (29): An illustration showing how natural deep eutectic solvents are extracted

Phytochemical component analysis and assessment of Brachychiton populneus's in vitro antioxidant capabilities

Phytonutrients display several health effects such as antibacterial, anti-inflammatory, anti-diabetic, anti-cancer and anti-hypertensive effects. Most of the secondary metabolites derived in herbal medicinal plants have the ability to alleviate diseases related to oxidative stress. Medicinal plants owe their antioxidant properties to the presence of organic compounds to a large extent.

It is proven that phytochemicals cannot be ignored in the production of pharmaceutical products, which shed light on their therapeutic value and makes it easy to apply and develop particular applications and formulations. Polyphenols possess great importance in pharmacology and therapy given their strong antioxidant properties, ability to neutralize free radicals, and inhibit lipid peroxidation; all these features have been highlighted in recent research on the topic **[286-297]**.

Terpenoids are a vital category of plant-derived chemicals, which have the potential to be utilized as a treatment of the metabolic disorders associated with obesity. Development of innovative pharmacological formulations is impossible without a good knowledge of the chemical constituents that are found in plants. Isolation methods, bioactive property assessments, and pharmacological barrier solutions have been used to a large extent to help in the development of better pharmaceutical therapies **[298- 305]**.

Medicinal plants and their constituents have the possibility of acting as antioxidants since they can combat reactive radicals to form radical chain reactions and are capable of donating electrons. Superoxide dismutase (SOD) and reduced glutathione (GSH) are examples of antioxidants that the body can be able to produce itself or obtain in the food they eat. Plants are a major source of exogenous antioxidants to be used by human beings. There are many plant species in the world with therapeutic qualities, and the majority of them have highly antioxidant effects **[306].**

The result of the lack of antioxidants can be oxidative stress which is excess of reactive oxygen species (ROS) and reactive nitrogen species (RNS). The continued oxidative stress may cause extreme harm to cells by inducing the processes of necrosis and apoptosis, which are some of the mechanisms that can be involved in the pathogenesis of many diseases. Oxidative stress is largely responsible in a wide variety of clinical disorders that involve the major vital organs of the body including liver, lungs, kidney, heart, brain, and others.

It has been found that ROS-mediated cellular damage can be attenuated and prevented successfully using antioxidant-enriching foods and medicinal herbs in the diet. More medicinal plants have been tested with antioxidative activity with the successes of natural therapeutics **[307, 308].**

The Kurrajong is a member of the Sterculaceae family and is scientifically known as Brachychiton populneus. This tree has a relatively short trunk and thick apex foliage and generally grows to a relatively modest or moderate size with a height of up to 20 meters. The genus has a highly diverse range of chemical constituents that are of interest in their antioxidant, antibacterial, and antidiabetic activities as alkaloids, flavonoids, terpenes, sterols and coumarins. Medicinal plants have a wide range of chemical constituents in terms of their polarity and chemical characteristics. The extraction of compounds using solvents with different polarities in phytochemistry is done. The difference in compound yields may manifest itself through the usage of different solvents in the extraction process as it was witnessed by Shah et al. As our findings showed, BPA was the most effective to produce the highest number of chemicals, then BPH, and lastly, BPE produced the least number of chemicals.

On the other hand, the hexane fraction of the Rumex hastatus roots produced the least amount as outlined by Sahreen et al. To determine the effectiveness of plant treatments, an initial qualitative screening procedure that will validate the presence of phytochemicals can be used to identify that. Based on a recent work, B. populneus has bioactive compounds, i.e., coumarins, terpenoids, flavonoids, tannins, alkaloids, phenols, saponins, quinones, phytosteroids, triterpenoids, vitamin C, phlobatannins, sterols, glycosides, and betacyanin, which play a role in its biological activity.

It has been shown that none of the conventional solvents could be used to separate the phytochemicals according to their polarity and hence the distribution of phytochemicals was spread out in varied fractions. This observation is consistent with the past studies. Nonetheless, due to the absence of the anthraquinones, anthocyanins, saponins, coumarins, and sterols in BPH, which means that the latter had lower solubility in n-hexane, the n-hexane solvent managed to isolate some phytochemicals **[309-311]**.

The quantitative analysis showed high levels of saponins, alkaloids, flavonoids, phenols, tannins and terpenoids in the fractions of B. populneus. These findings suggest that the aqueous solvent has the greatest concentration of total flavonoids, and ethyl acetate is the best solvent in extracting total phenolics and tannins. This polarity allowed the extraction of fractions based on a given treatment goal **[312]**.

Most substances in different categories have been demonstrated to have therapeutic advantages to plants. In addition to their anticancer and cytotoxic properties, the polyphenolic plant-derived chemical tannins are remarkably effective in the treatment of diarrhea, haemorrhage, viral infections, haemorrhoids, bacterial and fungal infections and parasitic diseases. Phenols and flavonoids are important in inhibiting cancer, inflammation and oxidative stress.

Alkaloids have also been indicated to have anticancer properties, and are thought to have impact on neurological diseases resembling Alzheimer. Saponins have the ability to combat bacteria, fungus and pests. Their existence validates the medicinal capabilities of the species of *B. populneus* **[313-320]**.

Various methods, which possess their own mechanism and kinetics, have been developed to determine the antioxidative properties of botanical compounds. These techniques measure plants with multitude of techniques before determining their antioxidant properties. Several antioxidant tests were conducted to determine the antioxidative capacity of polar-based raw extracts of the antioxidant properties of BPM, BPH, BPE, BPC, BPB, and BPA.

The DPPH assay was used to measure the capacity to scavenge free radicals of the B. populneus extract. This method is rapid, highly sensitive and can be used to identify the antioxidant power of plant extracts and compounds. At low concentrations, the stable dark violet powder with a nitrogen core called DPPH changes color to yellow. The color change is influenced by the antioxidant capacity of the raw extract in neutralizing the DPPH radical by hydrogen donation. The presence of phenolics and flavonoids increases the scavenging ability of plants significantly.

These substances have strong scavenging abilities, in that, they either donate electrons or hydrogen to stabilize DPPH radicals, and are typically extracted with polar solvents. The Board of Directors has completed and approved the proposed budget to be used in the next fiscal year. The budget is a strategy and well-calculated financial plan and distribution of resources that has been revised and taken into consideration.

Our funding is strategically planned to achieve our key strategic projects and objectives by the next year. A fair amount of effort has been put in ensuring the resources are utilized in the most efficient and economic manner. The budget also takes into account several other issues, including operational needs, market trends and legal needs. Forecasting of revenue in the coming year is done by use of market research and some performance measures.

An intensive sales and marketing plan has also been developed so as to achieve our revenue targets. The plan includes strategies of capturing new markets and increasing our customer base. Also, the client loyalty and retention will be enhanced by special marketing campaigns and customer interaction programs.

Cost conservation has been established in order to make sure that spending is within the budgetary constraints. A variety of cost-cutting and efficiency measures have been suggested in an attempt to reduce unnecessary expenditure and enhance on the general financial performance. Moreover, regular checks and evaluations of expenses will be carried out in order to find additional ways of cost optimisation and minimisation.

Through constant reviewing of expenditure, we shall be targeting long term financial sustainability and stability. Capital projects and infrastructure development have been well scheduled to ensure successful operation and to create opportunity to grow in the future.

The capital expenditure budget will contain funds to finance renovations, expansions, and other critical maintenance that will be necessary to maintain our business. These investments aim at increasing competitiveness, productivity and quality in the market. Human resource management is a key element to the budget since it is a source of training, development and retention programmes.

The organisational effectiveness is high due to employee development programs and performance management systems that are geared towards enhancement of skills and competencies. In addition, an attempt will be made to create a positive and encouraging workplace that facilitates the satisfaction of employees. The legal and regulatory criteria are of utmost importance in the budget planning process.

The budget structure has included compliance procedures to minimise risks and ensure that it meets the relevant laws and regulations. Careful compliance monitoring and reporting will be conducted to prevent any possible violation of the law or regulations, which might lead to the risks facing the company [321].

Also in the budget are the contingency plans and risk management, in case of unexpected events and emergencies. In order to detect and address the possible risks that may compromise the financial stability of the organisation, risk assessment methods and tools have been invented.

Proactive risk and uncertainty management are intended to help us protect both the resources and the reputation of the organisation in case of unexpected challenges. Overall, the budgeted proposal is a detailed and well thought-out financial strategy that attempts to maximise performance and competitiveness, as well as in the long-term sustainability [322].

We will also be able to reach our strategic goals and promote the growth and development in the future through careful financial planning and management.

Although none of the six fractions showed an IC50 value lower than that of the standard ascorbic acid, the current study found that the aqueous extract of B. populneus shown encouraging antioxidant activity against DPPH. Flavonoids and other active polyphenols are responsible for the strong association between IC50 values and TPC/TFC levels **[323- 328].**

The hydroxyl radical is well known for its extreme reactivity, ability to seriously damage phospholipids in cell membranes, and negative interactions with polyunsaturated fatty acids. Despite its brief existence, this radical is essential in starting chain reactions that may be harmful to cells. These radicals then react with deoxyribose to produce a red color. The abundance of active components in B. populneus that can scavenge hydroxyl radicals was strongly correlated with the total phenolic content (TPC) and total flavonoid content (TFC).

Our results are in line with earlier research by Majid et al., who found significant activity in extracts of ethyl acetate and ethyl acetate-water. The goal of the iron chelating test was to reduce the iron-ferrozine complex's color intensity by using plant extracts having scavenging properties that prevented the complex from forming. The Griess reagent was used to assess nitric oxide activity and identify the presence of nitrite ions. Nitrite ion formation can be inhibited by scavenging compounds that take up available oxygen. Our results agreed with those of Duenas et al. and Kilani et al. **[329–335].**

The mixture's bright yellow color turns pale milky as the linoleic acid hydroperoxides react with β-carotene. The strength of the antioxidant is indicated by the intensity of the yellow color; samples devoid of antioxidants show a sharp drop in absorbance. According to our research, the BPA fraction had the lowest IC50 value and showed a high correlation with the total flavonoid content (TFC) and total phenolic content (TPC). In the β-carotene bleaching test of aqueous extracts from Lamiaceae herbs, Triantaphyllou also noted notable antioxidant qualities **[336, 337].**

This assay produces green phosphate Mo (V) by converting Mo (VI) to Mo (V) with the use of antioxidant chemicals or plant extract. According to our research, B. populneus's aqueous fraction has potent antioxidant properties because of its high concentration of flavonoids and phenolic chemicals. There is a strong association between the total flavonoid and phenolic content of the plant extracts and the phosphomolybdenum assay. Jan et al. discovered increased phosphomolybdenum activity in the aqueous extract in a related investigation, which was strongly correlated with the total phenolic and flavonoid content **[338, 339].**

The potassium ferricyanide reduction technique was used to assess the efficacy of reducing power in B. populneus. By adding hydrogen, a chemical with antioxidant qualities in the sample converts iron (Fe^{+3}) to ferrous (Fe^{+2}), changing the reaction mixture's color from yellow to green. The brilliant green color seen during the test indicates the sample's great antioxidant capacity and reducing power.

At a concentration of 500 µg/ml, the BPA fraction showed the highest level of reducing power compared to ascorbic acid, followed by BPE, BPB, BPM, BPC, and BPH. Our findings are in line with a work by Sahreen et al. that demonstrated the superior antioxidant activity of Rumex hastatus methanol extract after butanol treatment. Genes linked to oxidative stress in the endoplasmic reticulum and inflammatory pathways in the liver were suppressed in rats exposed to carbon tetrachloride when BPM was used **[340, 341].**

Preparation of extract

The plant's aerial parts were purified to get rid of dust before being dried for many weeks in a shady area. In order to obtain a uniform particle size, the completely dried plant material was next ground into a fine powder and put through a 60-mesh filter in a Willy Mill. 1.2 kg of powdered aerial plant material and 3 liters of commercial methanol were combined for 48 hours at 25 °C to do the extraction. Whatman No. 1 filter paper was used in the filtration procedure.

Liquid-liquid partitioning was applied to a fraction of BPM that had been combined with distilled water. The range of solvents used included butanol (another polar solvent), ethyl acetate (a polar solvent), chloroform, and n-hexane (an apolar solvent).

After being separated, each solvent fraction was given the designations BPH (hexane fraction), BPC (chloroform fraction), BPE (ethyl acetate fraction), and BPB (butanol fraction). For possible pharmacological evaluations, each fraction was dehydrated, quantified, and stored.

Qualitative phytochemical analysis

In order to find significant phytochemical components such flavonoids, phenols, tannins, alkaloids, saponins, terpenoids, coumarins, anthocyanins, and anthraquinones, the methanol extract of B. populneus was thoroughly examined using qualitative screening techniques.

Assessment of phenols

Harborne's qualitative evaluation approach was the research methodology used in this study. Following a dosing of 1 mg, each sample was combined with 10% ferric chloride and 2 cc of distilled water. A green or blue hue shift was used to visually detect the presence of phenols **[342].**

Assessment of flavonoids

For the alkaline reagent assay, Trease and Evans' method called for mixing 1 mg of each sample with 1 ml of 2 N sodium hydroxide. The ensuing yellow color confirmed the presence of flavonoids. One milliliter of each extract was mixed with a few drops of FeCl3 solution for the FeCl3 test. The production of a deep red precipitate indicated the presence of flavonoids. **[343, 344].**

Assessment of coumarins

1 cc of 10% sodium hydroxide was used to react with each 1 mg sample. The presence of coumarins was revealed by the sample taking on a yellowish tinge. **[345].**

Assessment of saponins

Two milligrams of each sample and two milliliters of distilled water were combined in a test tube to start the process of creating froth using distilled water. The test samples were then forcefully stirred for around fifteen minutes. The samples under investigation contained saponins, as evidenced by the formation of a foamy layer. To conduct the olive oil emulsion test, 1 ml of each sample was put into a different test tube, and then 5–6 drops of olive oil were added. To create a stable frothy layer, the mixture was then aggressively stirred. The creation of an emulsion was seen as proof that saponins were present **[346].**

Assessment of tannins

For the FeCl3 test, 1 mg of each individual sample was mixed with 2 ml of 5% ferric chloride. Tannins were indicated by the emergence of a dark blue or greenish black color **[347, 348].**

Assessment of terpenoids

Two milliliters of chloroform and concentrated sulfuric acid were added to the plant specimens after each 0.5 mg sample was carefully placed into a test tube. The emergence of a distinct brown layer between the two extra layers in the test tube confirmed the presence of terpenoids. **[349].**

Assessment of anthraquinones

A 2% dilution of hydrochloric acid was added to one milligram of each sample. The appearance of a crimson tint provided conclusive proof that anthraquinone was present. **[350].**

Assessment of anthocyanin and betacyanins

After carefully placing each 1 milligram specimen into a test tube, 2 milliliters of 1 N sodium hydroxide were added. The test sample was heated for approximately ten minutes at 100 degrees Celsius. A bluish-green tint indicated the presence of anthocyanins, whereas a yellow tint indicated the presence of betacyanins **[351].**

Assessment of alkaloids

Mayer assessed each 2 ml sample by mixing it with strong hydrochloric acid using a specific reagent called Mayer's reagent. In the Hager's test, two milliliters of each plant extract were mixed with a little amount of Hager's reagent, a saturated picric acid solution. The presence of alkaloids in the specimen was demonstrated by the production of bright yellow precipitates. **[352, 353].**

Assessment of glycosides

In a scientific experiment, Keller Killanis mixed one milliliter of distinct plant extracts with one milliliter of glacial acetic acid and let them cool. The presence of glycosides in the extract was shown by the formation of a reddish-brown ring at the junction of the two layers **[354].**

Assessment of sterols

In the Salkowski test, 1 ml of concentrated H2SO4 is carefully added along the tube's sides after 2 ml of plant extract and 5 ml of chloroform have been combined. The presence of sterols is indicated by the lowest layer's red hue. **[355].**

Assessment of steroids and phytosteroids

One milliliter of the plant test specimen was mixed with one milliliter of chloroform and a tiny amount of strong sulfuric acid. Whereas the formation of a bluish-brown ring showed the presence of phytosteroids in the tested materials, the appearance of a brown ring indicated the presence of steroids.

Assessment of triterpenoids

1.5 milliliters of plant test samples were treated with Libermann-Buchard Reagent, a mixture of concentrated sulfuric acid and acetic anhydride.

Assessment of quinones

Each plant sample was mixed with 1 milliliter of concentrated sulfuric acid for a total volume of 1 milliliter. The presence of quinones in the sample was indicated by the appearance of a red tint.

Assessment of oils and resins

Plant samples had to be placed on filter paper in order to monitor the appearance of a transparent quality that would indicate the presence of oils and resins in the samples being tested. Several fractions of B. populneus were subjected to a quantitative spectrophotometric examination using recognized methods to quantify the main phytochemical components, such as phenols, flavonoids, and tannins. **[356]**

Total flavonoid contents (TFC)

In a test tube, 0.3 ml of plant sample, 0.15 ml of $NaNO_2$ (0.5 mol/l), 0.3 M $AlCl_3 \cdot 6H_2O$, and 3.4 ml of methanol (30%) were successively added to generate a reaction mixture. One milliliter of 1 M NaOH was added after a five-minute incubation period. The reaction mixture's optical density was then measured at a wavelength of 506 nm using rutin as a reference standard for comparisons across concentrations between 0 and 100 mg/ml. **[357].**

Quantification of flavonoids

The method described by Krishnaiah et al. was followed in the quantification of flavonoid content. In conclusion, a 100 mg plant sample was extracted many times using 80% aqueous methanol (10 ml) at room temperature, and then it was filtered through 125 mm Whatman-42 filter paper. The resultant filtrate was put in a crucible for further drying after being evaporated in a water bath to eliminate moisture. Until a stable weight was reached, the sample's weight was closely observed **[358-362].**

Quantification of terpenoids

After being immersed in alcohol, the 100 mg plant sample was left to stand at room temperature for a whole day. The sample was then extracted the following day, and petroleum ether was used to further treat the filtrate. The total terpenoids present in the sample were determined to be the extract that was obtained from the ether **[363, 364].**

Antioxidant capacity determination assays

Seven studies were conducted to quantify the antioxidant capacity and evaluate the ways in which different substances can reduce the effects of different free radicals. To assess their effectiveness, a number of substances, including gallic acid, rutin, ascorbic acid, and catechin, were dissolved in one milliliter of analytical methanol or DMSO at a concentration of one milligram per milliliter. After then, these solutions were gradually diluted to 1000, 500, 250, 125, 62, 31.25, and 15.62 μg/mL.

Hydroxyl radical scavenging assay

A technique based on studies by Halliwell and Gutteridge was used to assess the ability of plant extracts to neutralize hydroxyl free radicals. In this method, 500 μl of 2.8 mM 2-deoxyribose is mixed with 0.1 M EDTA, 200 μl of 100 mM ferric chloride, 100 μl of 200 mM H2O2, and 100 μl of each plant extract in a phosphate buffer (50 mM, pH 7.4). 100 μl of 300 mM ascorbic acid was added to start the reaction, which was then incubated for one hour at 37°C.

The reaction mixture was then heated for 15 minutes in a water bath and cooled after 1 ml of 2.8% TCA and 1 ml of TBA (1% w/v) in 50 mM NaOH were added. Measurements of optical density were made at 532 nm. The following formula was used to measure the plant extracts' ability to scavenge hydroxyl radicals: The formula {(1 - Absorbance of Sample) / Absorbance of Control} × 100 can be used to calculate the percentage of hydroxyl radical scavenging activity **[365- 370].**

Nitric oxide scavenging assay

Bhaskar and Balakrishnan developed a method for assessing the antioxidant qualities of plant specimens using the Griess reagent. Napthylenediamine (0.1%) in distilled water and sulphanilamide (1%) in phosphoric acid (5%) are equal parts of the Griess reagent. 100 µl of each plant sample was mixed with 100 µl of 10 mM sodium nitroprusside in saline phosphate buffer. Following a three-hour incubation time and spectrophotometric analysis at 546 nm using ascorbate as the positive control, 1 ml of Griess reagent was added to the reaction mixture. Equation 1 was used to determine the percentage of nitric oxide radical formation inhibition. **[371- 374]**

Chelating power assay

According to the technique outlined by Dastmalchi et al., the capacity of iron (II) to bind at many locations is thought to be responsible for the putative antioxidant qualities seen in plant samples. A 200 µl plant aliquot was combined with 900 µl of methanol and 100 µl of 2 mM $FeCl_2 \cdot 2H_2O$ for the experiment, which was then incubated for five minutes.

The reaction was then started by adding 400 µl of 5 mM ferrozine. After an extra ten minutes of incubation, the reaction mixture was examined using spectrophotometry at 562 nm, using EDTA as the standard reference. A certain equation was then used to determine the chelating capacity. **[375]**

β-Carotene bleaching assay

The plant's capability to bleach β-Carotene was evaluated using a methodology recommended by Elzaawely et al. The chloroform was then removed from the mixture using a vacuum, and 50 ml of distilled water was added, vigorously stirred to achieve a uniform emulsion of β-carotene linoleate.

Subsequently, 250 μl of the freshly prepared emulsion was mixed with 30 μl of each plant sample, and the optical density was measured at time 0 h at a wavelength of 470 nm. The reaction mixture was incubated at 45 °C for 2 h, and the final optical density was recorded. Catechin was used as a control in this analysis. The inhibition of β-carotene was determined by making slight modifications to the formula recommended by Mallet et al. **[376, 377]**

Reducing power assay

The process described by Landry et al. was employed in order to assess the reducing power activity. A solution comprising 2 ml of plant extract, 2 ml of 0.2 M phosphate buffer (pH 6.6), and 2 ml of potassium ferricyanide (10 mg/l) was prepared and allowed to incubate at a temperature of 50 °C for a duration of 20 minutes. Following this, 2 ml of trichloroacetic acid (TCA) (100 mg/l) was introduced into the mixture. A sample of the solution, measuring 2 ml, was then combined with 2 ml of distilled water and 0.4 ml of FeCl3 (0.1%) in a test tube. Gallic acid served as the standard for this particular analysis. The optical density was determined at a wavelength of 700 nm after 10 minutes. **[388]**

Phosphomolybdenum assay

According to Umamaheswari and Chatterjee's approach, the phosphomolybdenum test method was used to confirm the plant sample's antioxidant qualities. The resultant mixture was heated to 95 °C for 90 minutes in a water bath while being protected from light with silver foil. The combination was then allowed to cool to ambient temperature before being examined using spectrophotometry at 765 nm. In this test, ascorbic acid was the standard **[379]. Fig. 30**

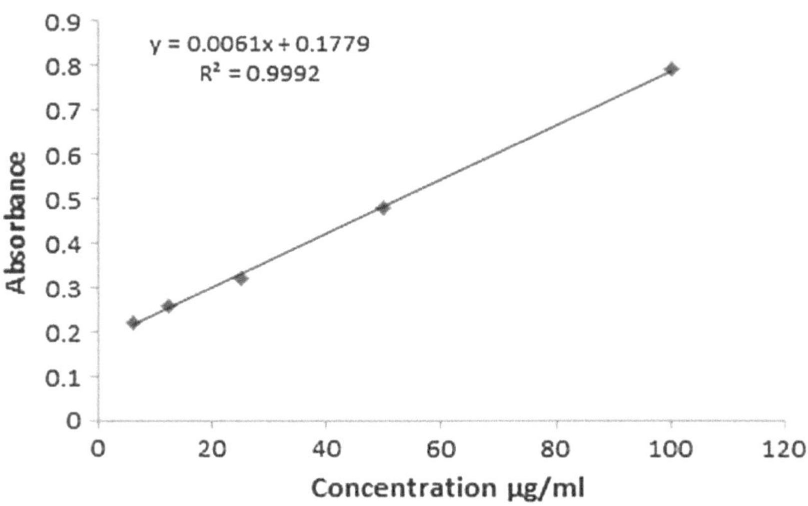

Fig (30): The regression line showing how gallic acid and total phenolic content are related

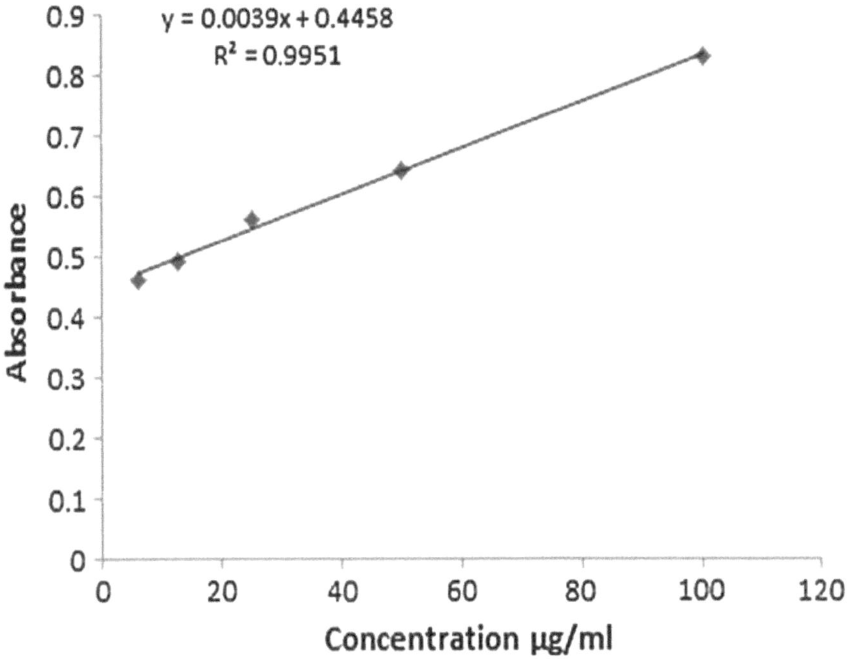

Fig. (31): The rutin regression line with respect to the total flavonoid content

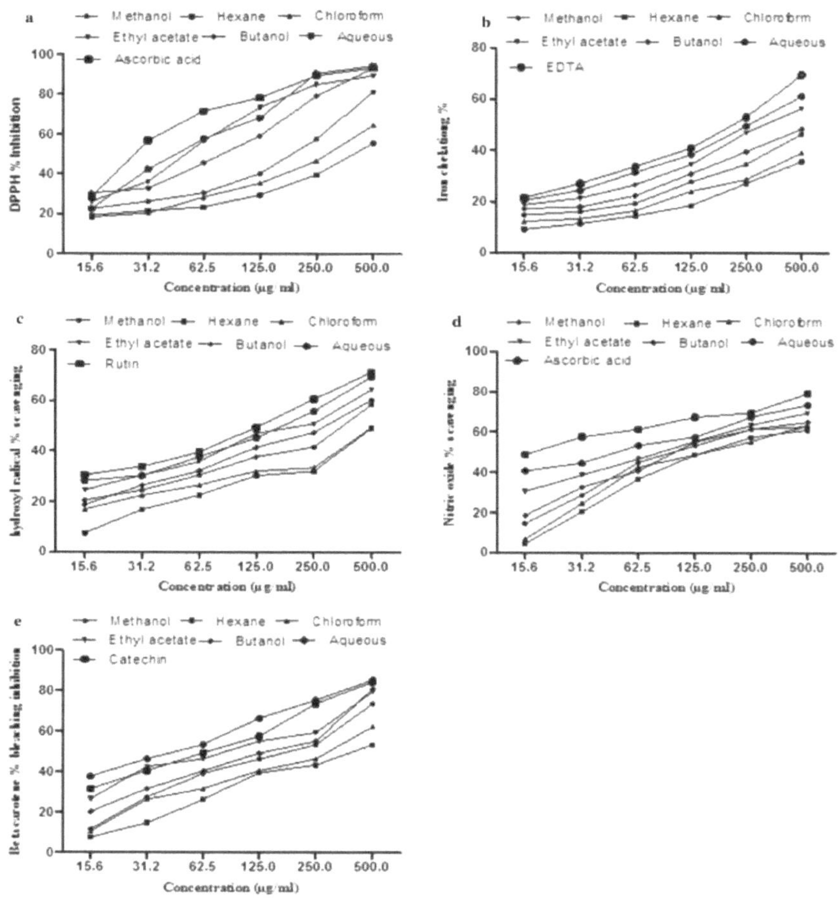

Fig. (32): DPPH inhibition, iron chelation, hydroxyl radical scavenging, nitric oxide scavenging, and β-carotene bleaching were all evaluated in these tests

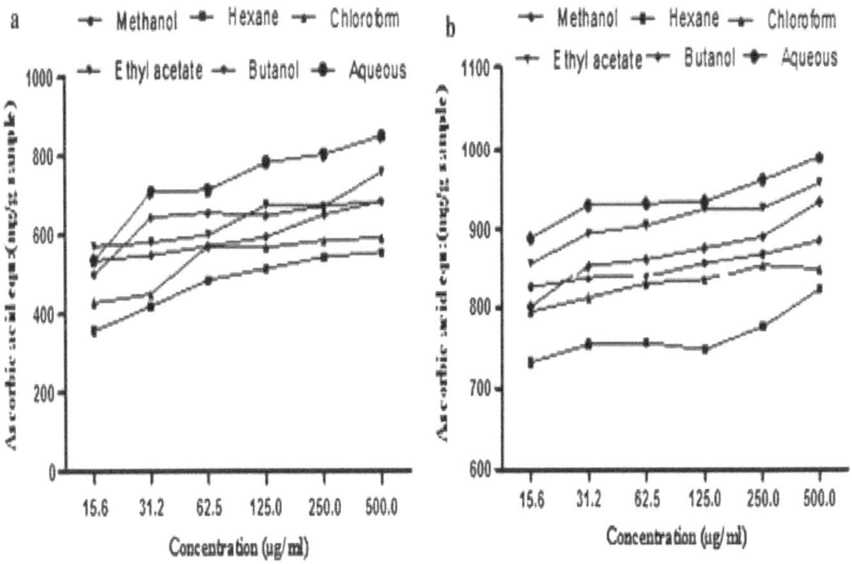

Fig. (33): The phosphomolybdate assay is used to measure the total antioxidant capacity. The reducing power assay of BPM and its constituent parts is evaluated.

Phytochemical screening

Despite the remarkable breakthroughs in contemporary medicine, infectious diseases caused by germs continue to be a huge threat to the world. The public's health is seriously threatened by these diseases, which are growing more prevalent and severe. This changing environment highlights the critical need to find novel, effective, and reasonably priced medications to treat infections, particularly in developing countries where infectious diseases account for half of all fatalities **[380- 385].**

The capacity of a variety of antimicrobial compounds derived from both natural and synthetic sources to fight illnesses has been acknowledged throughout history. However, only a few of these substances are readily available worldwide. The problems with the cost and accessibility of such therapies have become more complex due to the emergence of bacteria that are resistant to many drugs. Consequently, rates of illness, death, and healthcare expenditure have increased **[386, 387].**

Free radicals are instrumental in the development of numerous diseases. Reactive oxygen species (ROS) are constantly produced by redox enzymes in the body as they react with external substances under specific conditions. **[388-395]**

In a previous research conducted on ethnobotanical practices linked to the use of medicinal plants, several plants were identified for their frequent application in treating oral microbial diseases in the main city of the Democratic Republic of Congo. Specifically, Dysphania ambrosioides (L.) Mosyakin & Clemants, Ocimum gratissimum L., and Tetradenia riparia (Hochst.) For a variety of therapeutic purposes, Codd was commonly cited and frequently combined.

Numerous research has emphasized its many therapeutic advantages, such as its antibacterial, anesthetic, anti-inflammatory, and antipyretic properties. Furthermore, the plant extract has long been used to treat gastrointestinal parasites in both people and animals **[396- 400].**

It has been discovered that T. riparia extracts and essential oils exhibit a range of qualities, including antiviral, bioacaricidal, and antibacterial and antifungal activities. larvicidal, antimalarial, insecticidal, antiproliferative, and antioxidant qualities **[401- 404].**

Qualitative phytochemical screening

The components present in botanical extracts and their distribution are examined using the phytochemical screening process. This first step is crucial for finding bioactive substances and is crucial for the development of therapeutic interventions **[405- 410].**

Because of their well-known antioxidant properties, flavonoids are essential in preventing the growth and spread of malignancies. Terpenoids, on the other hand, exhibit a wide range of pharmacological characteristics, including antibacterial, anti-inflammatory, anticancer, and antioxidant qualities **[411- 415]**

Total phenolic and flavonoid content

The results showed that among the three, T. riparia had the highest total phenolic content (299.146 ± 0.143 mg GAE/g extract), followed by D. ambrosioides (155.602 ± 1.712 mg GAE/g extract) and O. gratissimum (153.597 ± 5.277 mg GAE/g extract) **[416, 417]**

Our findings marginally outperform those of Olamilosoye et al. (2018) and Panda et al. (2022). The date of plant harvest, soil acidity, drying techniques, geographic location, chemical makeup, or particular plant species or varieties used, as well as the extraction process used, could all contribute to this difference. The antioxidant, antimutagenic, and anti-carcinogenic qualities of phenolic substances are well known ability to modulate gene expression.

Flavonoids are bioactive constituents with a wide range of biological functions, including combating microbial infections, ulcers, arthritis, angiogenesis, and cancer, as well as inhibiting mitochondrial adhesion formation **[418-420]**.

UPLC analysis

Ultra-performance liquid chromatography-quadrupole time-of-flight mass spectrometry (UPLC-QTOF-MS) is a widely used technique for the detection of a broad spectrum of metabolites found in plants **[421- 423]. Fig. 36**

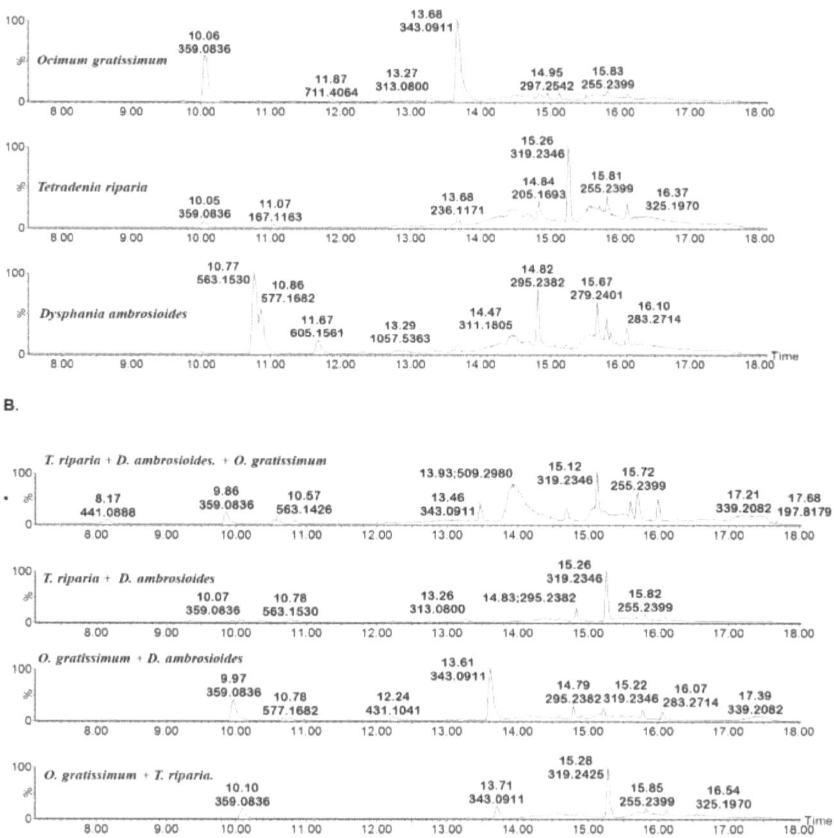

Fig. (33): ESI negative mode BPI chromatograms.

Antibacterial activity

These extracts showed reduced effectiveness of 2000 µg/mL against gram-negative bacteria such as Escherichia coli and Pseudomonas aeruginosa.

Gram-negative bacteria's outer membrane, which serves as a barrier to permeability and restricts the entry of numerous substances, including antimicrobial drugs, may be the cause of this reduced potency against them **[425, 426]**.

It is known that phenols, such as rosmarinic acid, can interfere with energy metabolism and cytoplasmic membrane function, which eventually affects nucleic acid synthesis. These substances have a wide variety of biological actions, such as antimicrobial, anti-aging, anti-cancer, anti-diabetic, and anti-depressant properties.

As a result, it is critical to evaluate the effects of mixing plant extracts, particularly as described by indigenous groups **[427-430]**.

Plant-Derived Natural Products

Oral cultural traditions have passed down the exact dosages and application methods of certain plants for specific medical problems, which have since been documented in traditional pharmacy writings. Pharmaceuticals made from medicinal plants are identified using a variety of academic disciplines and research techniques. Plant ecologists, botanists, ethnobotanists, and ethnopharmacologists frequently work together to identify and classify plants that may have therapeutic uses. **[431-436].**

The production of biotechnological pharmaceuticals, drugs, and therapies has been made easier by the conversion of botanical organisms into complex facilities that can synthesize natural therapeutic substances thanks to new technical developments.

Since morphine was first isolated from the Papaver somniferum plant in the early 9th century, the use of plants for therapeutic reasons has required the careful isolation of bioactive components. Additionally, current research endeavors have identified a plethora of other bioactive molecules derived from plants, which have undergone further refinement and commercialization as pharmaceutical therapies. [**437-440**].

The current study emphasizes the value of nature as a rich source of bioactive substances that aid in the creation of novel medications and treatments in the field of modern medicine. To standardize the usage of herbal treatments and identify important biomarkers for assessment, traditional drug discovery techniques have been applied. This gives medical practitioners a way to treat serious illnesses like diabetes, cancer, tuberculosis, asthma, influenza, coronary artery disease, and gastrointestinal disorders.

A viable, affordable, and secure substitute for traditional approaches that depend on microbial fermentation or animal cell cultures is the application of botanical pharmaceutical techniques in drug development. Therefore, drugs made from plant-based substances can provide patients with better and faster access to therapies **[441, 442].**

Historical Significance

Many different cultures around the world have used and acknowledged the therapeutic qualities of plants. In addition to enduring across time, these ancient traditions have had a major influence on the development of contemporary pharmacology and medical procedures. **[443- 447].**

A comprehensive understanding of this long-lasting relationship can be obtained by looking at significant accomplishments in the historical application of plant-derived therapies.

Healing techniques that were practiced by the Egyptians around 1500 BCE

Numerous contemporary herbal treatments and medical procedures have been impacted by their expertise and techniques. With more than 700 incantations and traditional healings that mainly rely on drawing, this document is regarded as one of the oldest medical manuscripts in existence **[448- 452].**

Chinese traditional herbal medicine dates back to ancient times

Traditional herbal treatment has been practiced for generations in China. Chinese herbal medicine is based on a vast understanding of many plant, mineral, and animal ingredients, many of which are still essential to contemporary TCM. TCM often combines different botanicals to have a synergistic effect, in contrast to Western medicine's focus on individual treatments. **[453- 457].**

Plant Collection

Botany and ethnobotany specialists must be involved in the early phases of pharmaceutical research and development in order to identify and gather plant species with promising therapeutic characteristics. Gathering the various beneficial chemicals found in plants is the first step towards identifying them. [**458, 459**].

Extraction

Depending on the characteristics and chemical makeup of the plant material, different methods may be used. Common techniques for separating chemicals **[460, 461].**

Supercritical fluid extraction is a widely used technique that uses carbon dioxide as a solvent under critical conditions, having both liquid and gas properties. **[462- 465].**

Isolation and Purification

The combination is put through purification and fractionation procedures to separate the active ingredients. Additionally, different methods like as crystallization and solvent partitioning could be used to refine the targeted compounds. [**466- 470**].

Bioassays

The next important step is to assess the compounds' pharmacological efficacy after they have been isolated and purified. The safety, effectiveness, and possible mechanisms of action of these drugs are assessed using a variety of assays, both in vitro and in vivo. On the other hand, in vivo experiments entail giving the substances to living things in order to learn more about their physiological and toxicological characteristics. **[471, 472].**

Structural Characterization

Understanding the characteristics and possible uses of molecules of interest in pharmaceutical research requires knowing their chemical makeup. **[473- 475].**

Biodiversity of Medicinal Plants

The term "biodiversity" refers to a wide variety of living things, including microorganisms, plants, animals, and the different environments they live in. It also relates to genetic makeup differences and the many ecosystems that result from these differences. Species diversity, ecological diversity, and genetic diversity are the three primary categories of biodiversity. [**476- 480**].

The vast range of plant species that can be found all over the world is referred to as plant biodiversity. Plants and animals cohabit in particular natural settings called "biotopes" to create a balanced ecosystem. With the exception of frigid areas and high mountain summits, most of the Earth's surface is naturally covered in plants. Temperature and geographic location are two examples of variables that greatly affect the composition of plant life **[481- 490].**

Oberholzeria etendekaensis, a novel species of succulent shrublet in a recently identified genus that is only found in Namibia and has a small population of only 30 known specimens, was another significant discovery. Furthermore, Brazil is known for having the greatest number of seed plants in the world, and knowledge of its varied plant life is still developing quickly [**491-495**].

The Place of Plants in the Traditional Pharmacopeia

Medicinal plants are used in traditional medicine all over the world to treat and prevent diseases in both human and animal populations. Furthermore, the significance of these plants for the advancement of world civilizations cannot be emphasized. **[496-500].**

There is a wealth of information on the therapeutic qualities of natural plants in almost every society on the planet. Additionally, the exchange of knowledge between civilizations has enhanced each group's pharmacopoeia by adding plants that are utilized by others to treat a variety of illnesses. [**501- 505**].

Herbal medicine is currently being used everywhere in the world. The growing acknowledgment of therapeutic plants, especially in developing nations where access to modern healthcare is restricted and medicinal plants are the main type of therapy available, is contributing to the continuously increasing economic relevance of herbal medicine.

These developing countries have many traits, including low levels of education, poor communication systems, a lack of resources, great distances between population centers, and pervasive poverty [**506- 510**].

The Role of Plants in Modern Medicine

Natural products continue to be a major focus in pharmaceutical research since conventional drug development methods often fail to deliver the wide range of chemical components required for treating disorders including metabolic and viral diseases [**511- 515**].

These organic substances have been and will remain essential to the creation of novel pharmaceutical therapies. Natural pharmaceuticals may be a safer alternative than drug metabolites derived from synthetic sources since they can cooperate with cells to achieve therapeutic benefits without causing negative side effects.

These essential characteristics are demonstrated by cellulose nanofibers generated from natural sources, alkaloids, flavonoids, and terpenoids. In order to survive in their environment, organisms have evolved specialized systems that have produced a vast diversity of chemical compounds that might serve as an inspiration for the development of novel medical treatments **[516- 520].**

Medicinal plants are the source of many recently created medications, demonstrating the wide range of use of plants in medicine, from simple preparations to complex molecules with distinct molecular structures. The potential therapeutic effects of these natural medicines, which have been an essential element of traditional medicine for generations, are currently being investigated scientifically in contemporary healthcare procedures.

Research is now being done on the possible uses of CBD in the treatment of ailments like epilepsy, anxiety, and chronic pain. The continuous importance of medicinal plants in the creation of innovative pharmaceuticals is highlighted by the approval of a number of new plant-based treatments as well as synthetic drugs using plant-based constituents. **[521- 526].**

Certain synthetic forms of delta-9-tetrahydrocannabinol, which is derived from Cannabis sativa L., have recently been approved in the United States for the treatment of chemotherapy-induced nausea. Additionally, cannabinoids are being investigated for their potential as antiasthmatics, antihypertensives, and powerful analgesics, as well as for the treatment of neurological disorders and glaucoma. **[527- 530].**

Conclusion

To identify the best extraction techniques, more comparative study is required, with an emphasis on comparing methods based on related principles.

Whereas the combination of O. gratissimum and D. ambrosioides shown additive effects, the decocted extracts of O. gratissimum and T. riparia demonstrated a synergistic antioxidant effect.

Furthermore, O. gratissimum and T. riparia demonstrated the greatest efficacy against Staphylococcus aureus, and their combination demonstrated further antibacterial benefits. The antibacterial activity was more noticeable in percolated extracts. These effects are thought to be caused by bioactive substances such xanthomicrol, rosmarinic acid, and other flavonoids.

In the past, natural substances derived from plants have been essential in producing therapeutic agents and acting as models for drug design, semisynthesis, and synthesis to treat a variety of diseases in both humans and animals. There are many chances to investigate the medicinal and other biological elements of hitherto undiscovered natural sources, as interest in creating herbal treatments with few adverse effects grows. Plant phytochemicals are refined in the field of drug development and discovery from plants to produce possible analogs with the required efficacy and safety.

Many cutting-edge techniques and technological developments have been created to support the selection, identification, isolation, characterisation, and biological assessment of natural components as medicinal chemists show a growing interest in creating medications based on natural chemicals. These novel strategies have the potential to overcome the technical difficulties involved in the creation of natural products as well as the barriers that arise in the investigation and manufacturing of novel natural medicines because of their complexity.

It is expected that new bioactive substances will be found in plants, which will eventually aid in the development of cutting-edge remedies for illnesses and microbial infections. In order to preserve and use these species for the benefit of future generations, it is imperative that endangered, threatened, and overexploited plant genetic resources be protected.

References

1. Germolec, D.R.; Shipkowski, K.A.; Frawley, R.P.; Evans, E. Markers of Inflammation. *Methods Mol. Biol.* **2018**, *1803*, 57–79.
2. Ferrucci, L.; Fabbri, E. Inflammageing: Chronic inflammation in ageing, cardiovascular disease, and frailty. *Nat. Rev. Cardiol.* **2018**, *15*, 505–522.
3. Zuo, L.; Prather, E.R.; Stetskiv, M.; Garrison, D.E.; Meade, J.R.; Peace, T.I.; Zhou, T. Inflammaging and Oxidative Stress in Human Diseases: From Molecular Mechanisms to Novel Treatments. *Int. J. Mol. Sci.* **2019**, *20*, 4472.
4. Kang, K.S. Phytochemical Constituents of Medicinal Plants for the Treatment of Chronic Inflammation. *Biomolecules* **2021**, *11*, 672.
5. Ajmal, S.; Shafqa, M.; Ajmal, L.; Younas, H.; Tasadduq, R.; Mahmood, N. Evaluation of Anti-cancer and Anti-proliferative Activity of Medicinal Plant Extracts (Saffron, Green Tea, Clove, Fenugreek) on Toll Like Receptors Pathway. *Nat. Prod. Sci.* **2022**, *28*, 121–129.
6. Moon, S.Y.; Kim, K.D.; Yoo, J.; Lee, J.H.; Hwangbo, C. Phytochemicals Targeting JAK–STAT Pathways in Inflammatory Bowel Disease: Insights from Animal Models. *Molecules* **2021**, *26*, 2824.
7. Kim, J.-H.; Lee, S.; Lee, M.-Y.; Shin, H.-K. Therapeutic effect of Soshiho-tang, a traditional herbal formula, on liver fibrosis or cirrhosis in animal models: A systematic review and meta-analysis. *J. Ethnopharmacol.* **2014**, *154*, 1–16.
8. Lee, J.-H.; Jo, E.H.; Lee, B.; Noh, H.M.; Park, S.; Lee, Y.-M.; Kim, D.-K.; Park, M.C. Soshiho-Tang, a traditional herbal medicine, alleviates atopic

dermatitis symptoms via regulation of inflammatory mediators. *Front. Pharmacol.* **2019**, *10*, 742.

9. Hopkins, A.L. Network pharmacology: The next paradigm in drug discovery. *Nat. Chem. Biol.* **2008**, *4*, 682–690.
10. Tarkang, P.A.; Appiah-Opong, R.; Ofori, M.F.; Ayong, L.S.; Nyarko, A.K. Application of multi-target phytotherapeutic concept in malaria drug discovery: A systems biology approach in biomarker identification. *Biomark. Res.* **2016**, *4*, 25.
11. Ren, J.L.; Zhang, A.H.; Kong, L.; Han, Y.; Yan, G.L.; Sun, H.; Wang, X.J. Analytical strategies for the discovery and validation of quality-markers of traditional Chinese medicine. *Phytomedicine* **2020**, *67*, 153165.
12. Kumar, A.; Kini, S.G.; Rathi, E. A recent appraisal of artificial intelligence and in silico ADMET prediction in the early stages of drug discovery. *Mini Rev. Med. Chem.* **2021**, *21*, 2788–2800.
13. Veiga, M.; Costa, E.M.; Silva, S.; Pintado, M. Impact of plant extracts upon human health: A review. *Crit. Rev. Food Sci. Nutr.* **2020**, *60*, 873–886.
14. Proestos, C. The benefits of plant extracts for human health. *Foods* **2020**, *9*, 1653.
15. Nathan, D.M. Long-term complications of diabetes mellitus. *N. Engl. J. Med.* **1993**, *328*, 1676–1685.
16. Ansari, P.; Akther, S.; Hannan, J.M.A.; Seidel, V.; Nujat, N.J.; Abdel-Wahab, Y.H. Pharmacologically active phytomolecules isolated from traditional antidiabetic plants and their therapeutic role for the management of diabetes mellitus. *Molecules* **2022**, *27*, 4278.
17. Kowalski, M.L.; Asero, R.; Bavbek, S.; Blanca, M.; Blanca-Lopez, N.; Bochenek, G.; Brockow, K.; Campo, P.; Celik, G.; Cernadas, J.; et al.

Classification and practical approach to the diagnosis and management of hypersensitivity to nonsteroidal anti-inflammatory drugs. *Allergy* **2013**, *68*, 1219–1232.

18. Rainsford, K. Anti-inflammatory drugs in the 21st century. *Sub-Cell. Biochem.* **2007**, *42*, 3–27.
19. Mohsen, S.; Dickinson, J.A.; Somayaji, R. Update on the adverse effects of antimicrobial therapies in community practice. *Can. Fam. Physician Med. Fam. Can.* **2020**, *66*, 651–659.
20. Basak, D.; Arrighi, S.; Darwiche, Y.; Deb, S. Comparison of anticancer drug toxicities: Paradigm shift in adverse effect profile. *Life* **2021**, *12*, 48.
21. Nurgali, K.; Jagoe, R.T.; Abalo, R. Adverse effects of cancer chemotherapy: Anything new to improve tolerance and reduce sequelae? *Front. Pharmacol.* **2018**, *9*, 245.
22. Ahmadiani, S.; Nikfar, S. Challenges of access to medicine and the responsibility of pharmaceutical companies: A legal perspective. *DARU J. Fac. Pharm. Tehran Univ. Med. Sci.* **2016**, *24*, 13.
23. Ramesh, P.; Okigbo, R.N. Effects of plants and medicinal plant combinations as anti-infectives. *Afr. J. Pharm. Pharmacol.* **2008**, *2*, 130–135.
24. Gibbons, S. An overview of plant extracts as potential therapeutics. *Expert Opin. Ther. Pat.* **2003**, *13*, 489–497.
25. Goyal, S.; Gupta, N.; Chatterjee, S.; Nimesh, S. Natural plant extracts as potential therapeutic agents for the treatment of cancer. *Curr. Top. Med. Chem.* **2017**, *17*, 96–106.

26. Pushpangadan, P.; George, V.; Ijinu, T.; Chithra, M.A. Ethnomedicine, health food and nutraceuticals-traditional wisdom of maternal and child health in India. *Edelweiss Appl. Sci. Technol.* **2018**, *2*, 113–117.
27. Zhu, Z.; Gui, Y.; Wang, L.; Wang, T.; Yang, Y.; Niu, Y.; Fu, D.; Wang, J.; Cui, T. Innovative development path of ethnomedicines: A case study. *Front. Med.* **2017**, *11*, 297–305.
28. Verma, S.; Singh, S.P. Current and future status of herbal medicines. *Vet. World* **2008**, *1*, 347.
29. Fazil, M.; Nikhat, S. Exploring new horizons in health care: A mechanistic review on the potential of Unani medicines in combating epidemics of infectious diseases. *Phytother. Res. PTR* **2021**, *35*, 2317–2335.
30. Singh, R.S.; Singh, A.; Kaur, H.; Batra, G.; Sarma, P.; Kaur, H.; Bhattacharyya, A.; Sharma, A.R.; Kumar, S.; Upadhyay, S.; et al. Promising traditional Indian medicinal plants for the management of novel Coronavirus disease: A systematic review. *Phytother. Res. PTR* **2021**, *35*, 4456–4484.
31. Živković, J.; Ilić, M.; Šavikin, K.; Zdunić, G.; Ilić, A.; Stojković, D. Traditional use of medicinal plants in South-Eastern Serbia (Pčinja District): Ethnopharmacological investigation on the current status and comparison with half a century old data. *Front. Pharmacol.* **2020**, *11*, 1020.
32. Yedjou, C.G.; Grigsby, J.; Mbemi, A.; Nelson, D.; Mildort, B.; Latinwo, L.; Tchounwou, P.B. The management of diabetes mellitus using medicinal plants and vitamins. *Int. J. Mol. Sci.* **2023**, *24*, 9085.
33. Firenzuoli, F.; Gori, L. European traditional medicine–international congress–introductory statement. *Evid.-Based Complement. Altern. Med. eCAM* **2007**, *4* (Suppl. 1), 3–4.

34. Ansari, P.; Flatt, P.R.; Harriott, P.; Hannan, J.M.A.; Abdel-Wahab, Y.H. Identification of multiple pancreatic and extra-pancreatic pathways underlying the glucose-lowering actions of *Acacia arabica* Bark in type-2 diabetes and isolation of active phytoconstituents. *Plants* **2021**, *10*, 1190.
35. Hegazy, G.A.; Alnoury, A.M.; Gad, H.G. The role of *Acacia arabica* extract as an antidiabetic, antihyperlipidemic, and antioxidant in streptozotocin-induced diabetic rats. *Saudi Med. J.* **2013**, *34*, 727–733.
36. Matheka, D.M.; Alkizim, F.O. Complementary and alternative medicine for type 2 diabetes mellitus: Role of medicinal herbs. *J. Diabetes Endocrinol.* **2012**, *3*, 44–56.
37. Ojieh, A.E.; Adegor, E.C.; Okolo, A.C.; Lawrence, E.O.; Njoku, I.P.; Onyekpe, C.U. Hypoglycemic and hypolipidaemic effect of allium cepa in streptozotocin-induced diabetes. *Int. J. Sci. Eng.* **2015**, *6*, 23–29
38. Eyo, J.E.; Ozougwu, J.C.; Echi, P.C. Hypoglycaemic effects of *Allium cepa*, *Allium sativum* and *Zingiber officinale* aqueous extracts on alloxan-induced diabetic Rattus novergicus. *Med. J. Islam. World Acad. Sci.* **2011**, *19*, 121–126.
39. Jawonisi, I.O.; Adoga, G.I. Hypoglycaemic and hypolipidaemic effect of extract of *Lantana camara* Linn. leaf on alloxan diabetic rats. *J. Nat. Sci. Res.* **2015**, *5*, 6–10.
40. Venkatesh, S.; Latha, R.; Anaswara, R.N.; Jincy, T.C.; Muhammed Shibli, P.C.; Suresh, A. Anti-hyperglycemic and anti-oxidant activities of ethanolic extract of *Lantana camara* leaves. *Int. J. Front. Life Sci. Res.* **2021**, *1*, 5–15.
41. Bobson, P.G.M.; Afangideh, E.U.; Okon, O.E.; Akpan, M.O.; Tom, E.J.; Usen, R.F. Effect of Ethanol Leaf Extract of *Lantana camara* on Fasting Blood Glucose, Body Weight and Kidney Function Indices of Alloxan-

Induced Diabetic Albino Wistar Rats. *Asian J. Biochem. Genet. Mol. Biol.* **2024**, *16*, 89–96.

42. Jiang, S.; Xu, L.; Xu, Y.; Guo, Y.; Wei, L.; Li, X.; Song, W. Antidiabetic effect of *Momordica charantia* saponins in rats induced by high-fat diet combined with STZ. *Electron. J. Biotechnol.* **2020**, *43*, 41–47.
43. Ansari, P.; Khan, J.T.; Soultana, M.; Hunter, L.; Chowdhury, S.; Priyanka, S.K.; Paul, S.R.; Flatt, P.R.; Abdel-Wahab, Y.H. Insulin secretory actions of polyphenols of *Momordica charantia* regulate glucose homeostasis in alloxan-induced type 2 diabetic rats. *RPS Pharm. Pharmacol. Rep.* **2024**, *3*, rqae005.
44. Abas, R.; Othman, F.; Thent, Z.C. Protective Effect of *Momordica charantia* Fruit Extract on Hyperglycaemia-Induced Cardiac Fibrosis. *Oxidative Med. Cell. Longev.* **2014**, *2014*, 429060.
45. Tariq, A.; Sadia, S.; Pan, K.; Ullah, I.; Mussarat, S.; Sun, F.; Abiodun, O.O.; Batbaatar, A.; Li, Z.; Song, D.; et al. A systematic review on ethnomedicines of anti-cancer plants. *Phytother. Res.* **2017**, *31*, 202–264
46. Bharti, S.K.; Krishnan, S.; Kumar, A.; Kumar, A. Antidiabetic phytoconstituents and their mode of action on metabolic pathways. *Ther. Adv. Endocrinol. Metab.* **2018**, *9*, 81–100.
47. Mahapatra, A.D.; Bhowmik, P.; Banerjee, A.; Das, A.; Ojha, D.; Chattopadhyay, D. Ethnomedicinal wisdom: An approach for antiviral drug development. In *New Look to Phytomedicine*; Academic Press: Cambridge, MA, USA, 2019; pp. 35–61.
48. Vaou, N.; Stavropoulou, E.; Voidarou, C.; Tsigalou, C.; Bezirtzoglou, E. Towards advances in medicinal plant antimicrobial activity: A review study on challenges and future perspectives. *Microorganisms* **2021**, *9*, 2041.

49. Dabur, R.; Gupta, A.; Mandal, T.K.; Singh, D.D.; Bajpai, V.; Gurav, A.M.; Lavekar, G.S. Antimicrobial activity of some Indian medicinal plants. *Afr. J. Tradit. Complement. Altern. Med. AJTCAM* **2007**, *4*, 313–318.
50. Ngezahayo, J.; Ribeiro, S.O.; Fontaine, V.; Hari, L.; Stévigny, C.; Duez, P. In vitro study of five herbs used against microbial infections in Burundi. *Phytother. Res. PTR* **2017**, *31*, 1571–1578.
51. Kamyab, R.; Namdar, H.; Torbati, M.; Ghojazadeh, M.; Araj-Khodaei, M.; Fazljou, S.M.B. Medicinal plants in the treatment of hypertension: A review. *Adv. Pharm. Bull.* **2021**, *11*, 601–617.
52. Shin, S.A.; Joo, B.J.; Lee, J.S.; Ryu, G.; Han, M.; Kim, W.Y.; Park, H.H.; Lee, J.H.; Lee, C.S. Phytochemicals as anti-inflammatory agents in animal models of prevalent inflammatory diseases. *Molecules* **2020**, *25*, 5932.
53. Leitzmann, C. Characteristics and health benefits of phytochemicals. *Forsch. Komplementärmedizin* **2016**, *23*, 69–74.
54. Khameneh, B.; Eskin, N.M.; Iranshahy, M.; Fazly Bazzaz, B.S. Phytochemicals: A promising weapon in the arsenal against antibiotic-resistant bacteria. *Antibiotics* **2021**, *10*, 1044.
55. Dehelean, C.A.; Marcovici, I.; Soica, C.; Mioc, M.; Coricovac, D.; Iurciuc, S.; Cretu, O.M.; Pinzaru, I. Plant-derived anticancer compounds as new perspectives in drug discovery and alternative therapy. *Molecules* **2021**, *26*, 1109.
56. Bailes, B.K. Diabetes mellitus and its chronic complications. *AORN J.* **2002**, *76*, 266–286.
57. Tomic, D.; Shaw, J.E.; Magliano, D.J. The burden and risks of emerging complications of diabetes mellitus. *Nat. Rev. Endocrinol.* **2022**, *18*, 525–539.

58. Rena, G.; Hardie, D.G.; Pearson, E.R. The mechanisms of action of metformin. *Diabetologia* **2017**, *60*, 1577–1585.
59. El-Saber Batiha, G.; Magdy Beshbishy, A.; G. Wasef, L.; Elewa, Y.H.; A Al-Sagan, A.; Abd El-Hack, M.E.; Taha, A.E.; M Abd-Elhakim, Y.; Prasad Devkota, H. Chemical constituents and pharmacological activities of garlic (*Allium sativum* L.): A review. *Nutrients* **2020**, *12*, 872.
60. Sato, M.; Dehvari, N.; Öberg, A.I.; Dallner, O.S.; Sandström, A.L.; Olsen, J.M.; Csikasz, R.I.; Summers, R.J.; Hutchinson, D.S.; Bengtsson, T. Improving type 2 diabetes through a distinct adrenergic signaling pathway involving mTORC2 that mediates glucose uptake in skeletal muscle. *Diabetes* **2014**, *63*, 4115–4129.
61. Nazarian-Samani, Z.; Sewell, R.D.; Lorigooini, Z.; Rafieian-Kopaei, M. Medicinal plants with multiple effects on diabetes mellitus and its complications: A systematic review. *Curr. Diabetes Rep.* **2018**, *18*, 72.
62. Bray, F.; Laversanne, M.; Sung, H.; Ferlay, J.; Siegel, R.L.; Soerjomataram, I.; Jemal, A. Global cancer statistics 2022: GLOBOCAN estimates of incidence and mortality worldwide for 36 cancers in 185 countries. *CA Cancer J. Clin.* **2024**, *74*, 229–263.
63. Prakash, O.; Kumar, A.; Kumar, P.; Ajeet. Anticancer potential of plants and natural products. *Am. J. Pharmacol. Sci.* **2013**, *1*, 104–115.
64. Choudhari, A.S.; Mandave, P.C.; Deshpande, M.; Ranjekar, P.; Prakash, O. Phytochemicals in cancer treatment: From preclinical studies to clinical practice. *Front. Pharmacol.* **2020**, *10*, 1614.
65. Pham, H.N.T.; Vuong, Q.V.; Bowyer, M.C.; Scarlett, C.J. Phytochemicals derived from *Catharanthus roseus* and their health benefits. *Technologies* **2020**, *8*, 80.

66. Fuloria, S.; Mehta, J.; Chandel, A.; Sekar, M.; Rani, N.N.I.M.; Begum, M.Y.; Subramaniyan, V.; Chidambaram, K.; Thangavelu, L.; Nordin, R.; et al. A comprehensive review on the therapeutic potential of *Curcuma longa* Linn. in relation to its major active constituent curcumin. *Front. Pharmacol.* **2022**, *13*, 820806.
67. Ranjan, A.; Ramachandran, S.; Gupta, N.; Kaushik, I.; Wright, S.; Srivastava, S.; Prasad, S.; Srivastava, S.K. Role of phytochemicals in cancer prevention. *Int. J. Mol. Sci.* **2019**, *20*, 4981.
68. Adico, M.D.; Bayala, B.; Zoure, A.A.; Lagarde, A.; Bazie, J.T.; Traore, L.; Buñay, J.; Yonli, A.T.; Djigma, F.; Bambara, H.A.; et al. In vitro activities and mechanisms of action of anti-cancer molecules from African medicinal plants: A systematic review. *Am. J. Cancer Res.* **2024**, *14*, 1376–1401.
69. Giordano, A.; Tommonaro, G. Curcumin and cancer. *Nutrients* **2019**, *11*, 2376.
70. Shaito, A.; Thuan, D.T.B.; Phu, H.T.; Nguyen, T.H.D.; Hasan, H.; Halabi, S.; Abdelhady, S.; Nasrallah, G.K.; Eid, A.H.; Pintus, G. Herbal medicine for cardiovascular diseases: Efficacy, mechanisms, and safety. *Front. Pharmacol.* **2020**, *11*, 422.
71. Chakraborty, A.J.; Uddin, T.M.; Matin Zidan, B.R.; Mitra, S.; Das, R.; Nainu, F.; Dhama, K.; Roy, A.; Hossain, M.J.; Khusro, A.; et al. *Allium cepa*: A treasure of bioactive phytochemicals with prospective health benefits. *Evid.-Based Complement. Altern. Med. Ecam* **2022**, *2022*, 4586318.
72. Ranjha, M.M.A.N.; Shafique, B.; Wang, L.; Irfan, S.; Safdar, M.N.; Murtaza, M.A.; Nadeem, M.; Mahmood, S.; Mueen-ud-Din, G.; Nadeem, H.R. A comprehensive review on phytochemistry, bioactivity and medicinal

value of bioactive compounds of pomegranate (*Punica granatum*). *Adv. Tradit. Med.* **2021**, *23*, 37–57.

73. Hossen, I.; Hua, W.; Ting, L.; Mehmood, A.; Jingyi, S.; Duoxia, X.; Yanping, C.; Hongqing, W.; Zhipeng, G.; Kaiqi, Z.; et al. Phytochemicals and inflammatory bowel disease: A review. *Crit. Rev. Food Sci. Nutr.* **2022**, *60*, 1321–1345.
74. Kumar, V.; Van Staden, J. A Review of Swertia chirayita (Gentianaceae) as a Traditional Medicinal Plant. *Front. Pharmacol.* **2016**, *6*, 308.
75. Sharifi-Rad, J.; Dey, A.; Koirala, N.; Shaheen, S.; El Omari, N.; Salehi, B.; Goloshvili, T.; Cirone Silva, N.C.; Bouyahya, A.; Vitalini, S.; et al. Cinnamomum species: Bridging phytochemistry knowledge, pharmacological properties and toxicological safety for health benefits. *Front. Pharmacol.* **2021**, *12*, 600139.
76. Maksoud, S.; Abdel-Massih, R.M.; Rajha, H.N.; Louka, N.; Chemat, F.; Barba, F.J.; Debs, E. *Citrus aurantium* L. active constituents, biological effects and extraction methods. an updated review. *Molecules* **2021**, *26*, 5832.
77. Klimek-Szczykutowicz, M.; Szopa, A.; Ekiert, H. *Citrus limon* (Lemon) phenomenon—A review of the chemistry, pharmacological properties, applications in the modern pharmaceutical, food, and cosmetics industries, and biotechnological studies. *Plants* **2020**, *9*, 119.
78. Liu, Y.; Zhang, W.; Xu, C.; Li, X. Biological activities of extracts from loquat (*Eriobotrya japonica* Lindl.): A review. *Int. J. Mol. Sci.* **2016**, *17*, 1983.

79. Tiwari, P.; Mishra, B.N.; Sangwan, N.S. Phytochemical and pharmacological properties of *Gymnema sylvestre*: An important medicinal plant. *BioMed Res. Int.* **2014**, *2014*, 830285.
80. Reddy, N.M. *Lantana camara* Linn. chemical constituents and medicinal properties: A review. *Sch. Acad. J. Pharm.* **2013**, *2*, 445–448.
81. Ajijolakewu, K.A.; Ayoola, A.S.; Agbabiaka, T.O.; Zakariyah, F.R.; Ahmed, N.R.; Oyedele, O.J.; Sani, A. A review of the ethnomedicinal, antimicrobial, and phytochemical properties of *Musa paradisiaca* (plantain). *Bull. Natl. Res. Cent.* **2021**, *45*, 86.
82. Zulkurnain, E.I.; Ramli, S.; Ali, A.A.; James, R.J.; Kamarazaman, I.S.; Halim, H. The Phytochemical and Pharmacological Effects of *Hibiscus rosa-sinensis*: A Review. *Int. J. Pharm. Investig.* **2023**, *13*, 422–431.
83. Saleem, S.; Muhammad, G.; Hussain, M.A.; Altaf, M.; Bukhari, S.N.A. *Withania somnifera* L.: Insights into the phytochemical profile, therapeutic potential, clinical trials, and future prospective. *Iran. J. Basic Med. Sci.* **2020**, *23*, 1501–1526.
84. Saravanan, S.; Hari, R.; Sekar, K. Anti-proliferative potentials of Aconitum heterophyllum Root Extract in Human Breast cancer (MDA-MB-231) cell lines-Genetic and Antioxidant enzyme approach. *Avicenna J. Med. Biotechnol.* **2023**, *15*, 188–195.
85. Wang, H.; Chen, Y.; Wang, L.; Liu, Q.; Yang, S.; Wang, C. Advancing Herbal Medicine: Enhancing Product Quality and Safety through Robust Quality Control Practices. *Front. Pharmacol.* **2023**, *14*, 1265178.
86. Inchingolo, A.D.; Inchingolo, A.M.; Malcangi, G.; Avantario, P.; Azzollini, D.; Buongiorno, S.; Viapiano, F.; Campanelli, M.; Ciocia, A.M.; De Leonardis, N.; et al. Effects of Resveratrol, Curcumin and Quercetin

Supplementation on Bone Metabolism—A Systematic Review. *Nutrients* **2022**, *14*, 3519.

87. El-Saadony, M.T.; Yang, T.; Korma, S.A.; Sitohy, M.; Abd El-Mageed, T.A.; Selim, S.; Al Jaouni, S.K.; Salem, H.M.; Mahmmod, Y.; Soliman, S.M.; et al. Impacts of Turmeric and Its Principal Bioactive Curcumin on Human Health: Pharmaceutical, Medicinal, and Food Applications: A Comprehensive Review. *Front. Nutr.* **2023**, *9*, 1040259.
88. Tabanelli, R.; Brogi, S.; Calderone, V. Improving Curcumin Bioavailability: Current Strategies and Future Perspectives. *Pharmaceutics* **2021**, *13*, 1715.
89. Asma, S.T.; Acaroz, U.; Imre, K.; Morar, A.; Shah, S.R.A.; Hussain, S.Z.; Arslan-Acaroz, D.; Demirbas, H.; Hajrulai-Musliu, Z.; Istanbullugil, F.R.; et al. Natural Products/Bioactive Compounds as a Source of Anticancer Drugs. *Cancers* **2022**, *14*, 6203.
90. Das, S.; Dey, M.K.; Devireddy, R.; Gartia, M.R. Biomarkers in Cancer Detection, Diagnosis, and Prognosis. *Sensors* **2024**, *24*, 37.
91. Khan, S.R.; Al Rijjal, D.; Piro, A.; Wheeler, M.B. Integration of AI and Traditional Medicine in Drug Discovery. *Drug Discov. Today* **2021**, *26*, 982–992.
92. Sanches, P.H.G.; de Melo, N.C.; Porcari, A.M.; de Carvalho, L.M. Integrating Molecular Perspectives: Strategies for Comprehensive Multi-Omics Integrative Data Analysis and Machine Learning Applications in Transcriptomics, Proteomics, and Metabolomics. *Biology* **2024**, *13*, 848.
93. Jendoubi, T. Approaches to Integrating Metabolomics and Multi-Omics Data: A Primer. *Metabolites* **2021**, *11*, 184.
94. Sharifi-Rad, J.; Herrera-Bravo, J.; Semwal, P.; Painuli, S.; Badoni, H.; Ezzat, S.M.; Farid, M.M.; Merghany, R.M.; Aborehab, N.M.; Salem, M.A.;

et al. *Artemisia* spp.: An Update on Its Chemical Composition, Pharmacological and Toxicological Profiles. *Oxidative Med. Cell. Longev.* **2022**, *2022*, 5628601.

95. Kumar KM, Asish G, Sabu M, Balachandran I. Significance of gingers (Zingiberaceae) in Indian system of medicine—ayurveda: an overview. Anc Sci Life. 2013;32:253. https://doi.org/10.4103/0257-7941.131989.

96. Perera DN, Hewavitharana GG, Navaratne SB. Determination of physicochemical and functional properties of coconut oil by incorporating bioactive compounds in selected spices. J Lipids. 2020;2020:1–11. https://doi.org/10.1155/2020/8853940.

97. Prasad S, Tyagi AK. Ginger and its constituents: role in prevention and treatment of gastrointestinal cancer. Gastroenterol Res Pract. 2015;2015:1–11. https://doi.org/10.1155/2015/142979.

98. Rahmani AH, Al SFM, Aly SM. Active ingredients of ginger as potential candidates in the prevention and treatment of diseases via modulation of biological activities. Int J Physiol Pathophysiol Pharmacol. 2014;6:125–36.

99. Unuofin JO, Masuku NP, Paimo OK, Lebelo SL. Ginger from farmyard to town: nutritional and pharmacological applications. Front Pharmacol. 2021. https://doi.org/10.3389/fphar.2021.779352.

100. Mashhadi NS, Ghiasvand R, Askari G, et al. Anti-oxidative and anti-inflammatory effects of ginger in health and physical activity: review of current evidence. Int J Prev Med. 2013;4:S36-42.

101. Ajanaku CO, Ademosun OT, Atohengbe PO, et al. Functional bioactive compounds in ginger, turmeric, and garlic. Front Nutr. 2022. https://doi.org/10.3389/fnut.2022.1012023.

102. Stephen Lansing J, Cox MP, de Vet TA, et al. An ongoing Austronesian expansion in Island Southeast Asia. J Anthropol Archaeol. 2011;30:262–72. https://doi.org/10.1016/j.jaa.2011.06.004.
103. Arslan A, Aygun YZ, Turkmen M, et al. Combining non-destructive devices and multivariate analysis as a tool to quantify the fatty acid profiles of linseed genotypes. Talanta. 2025;281: 126798. https://doi.org/10.1016/j.talanta.2024.126798.
104. Wang H. Introductory chapter: studies on ginger. In: ginger cultivation and its antimicrobial and pharmacological potentials. IntechOpen. 2020.
105. Atashpour S, Kargar Jahromi H, Kargar Jahromi Z, Maleknasab M. Comparison of the effects of Ginger extract with clomiphene citrate on sex hormones in rats with polycystic ovarian syndrome. Int J Reprod Biomed. 2017;15:561–8.
106. Arslan A, Alibaş İ. Assessing the effects of different drying methods and minimal processing on the sustainability of the organic food quality. Innov Food Sci Emerg Technol. 2024;94: 103681. https://doi.org/10.1016/j.ifset.2024.103681.
107. Yang Z, Guo Z, Yan J, Xie J. Nutritional components, phytochemical compositions, biological properties, and potential food applications of ginger (Zingiber officinale): a comprehensive review. J Food Compos Anal. 2024;128: 106057. https://doi.org/10.1016/j.jfca.2024.106057.
108. Ajayi OB, Akomolafe SF, Akinyemi FT. Food value of two varieties of ginger (Zingiber officinale) commonly consumed in Nigeria. ISRN Nutr. 2013;2013:1–5. https://doi.org/10.5402/2013/359727.
109. Khandouzi N, Shidfar F, Rajab A, et al. The effects of ginger on fasting blood sugar, hemoglobin a1c, apolipoprotein B, apolipoprotein a-I and

malondialdehyde in type 2 diabetic patients. Iran J Pharm Res IJPR. 2015;14:131–40.

110. Nwosu LC, Edo GI, Özgör E. The phytochemical, proximate, pharmacological, GC-MS analysis of Cyperus esculentus (Tiger nut): a fully validated approach in health, food and nutrition. Food Biosci. 2022;46: 101551. https://doi.org/10.1016/j.fbio.2022.101551.

111. Shaukat MN, Nazir A, Fallico B. Ginger bioactives: a comprehensive review of health benefits and potential food applications. Antioxidants. 2023;12:2015. https://doi.org/10.3390/antiox12112015.

112. Edo GI. Antibacterial, phytochemical and GC-MS analysis of Thevetia peruviana extracts: an approach in drug formulation. Nat Resour Hum Heal. 2022;2:418–26. https://doi.org/10.53365/nrfhh/146543.

113. Hassan F, Edo GI, Nwosu LC, et al. An inventory of medicinal plants used as sedative, analgesic and blood tonic in Abeokuta, Ogun state, Nigeria. Acta Ecol Sin. 2023;43:459–68. https://doi.org/10.1016/j.chnaes.2021.11.003.

114. Akpoghelie PO, Edo GI, Akhayere E. Proximate and nutritional composition of beer produced from malted sorghum blended with yellow cassava. Biocatal Agric Biotechnol. 2022;45: 102535. https://doi.org/10.1016/j.bcab.2022.102535.

115. Aderonke Otunola G, Jide Afolayan A. A Review of the Antidiabetic Activities of Ginger. In: Ginger Cultivation and Its Antimicrobial and Pharmacological Potentials. IntechOpen. 2020.

116. Jikah AN, Edo GI. Moringa oleifera: a valuable insight into recent advances in medicinal uses and pharmacological activities. J Sci Food Agric. 2023. https://doi.org/10.1002/jsfa.12892.

117. Edo GI, Ugbune U, Onoharigho FO, et al. Antioxidant activities of reissantia indica willd. (mopane paddle-pod) and nephroprotective effect on paracetamol-induced nephrotoxicity in male wistar rats. Nutrire. 2023;48:26. https://doi.org/10.1186/s41110-023-00214-x.

118. Edo GI, Ugbune U, Onoharigho FO, et al. Investigation of the metal complexes and bioactive compound formed by coordination of bioactive phytochemical from ginger (Zingiber officinale) extracts to metal ions. Food Chem Adv. 2023;3: 100337. https://doi.org/10.1016/j.focha.2023.100337.

119. Edo GI, Samuel PO, Jikah AN, et al. Proximate composition and health benefit of Roselle leaf (Hibiscus sabdariffa). Insight on food and health benefits. Food Chem Adv. 2023;3: 100437. https://doi.org/10.1016/j.focha.2023.100437.

120. Edo GI, Samuel PO, Jikah AN, et al. Biological and bioactive components of bitter leaf (Vernonia amygdalina leaf): insight on health and nutritional benefits. A review Food Chem Adv. 2023;3: 100488. https://doi.org/10.1016/j.focha.2023.100488.

121. Edo GI, Ugbune U, Ezekiel GO, et al. Cyperus esculentus (tiger nut): its application in agriculture, food, health and nutrition. A review. Vegetos. 2023. https://doi.org/10.1007/s42535-023-00672-8.

122. Oršolić N, Jazvinšćak Jembrek M. Molecular and cellular mechanisms of propolis and its polyphenolic compounds against cancer. Int J Mol Sci. 2022;23:10479. https://doi.org/10.3390/ijms231810479.

123. Semwal RB, Semwal DK, Combrinck S, Viljoen AM. Gingerols and shogaols: important nutraceutical principles from ginger. Phytochemistry. 2015;117:554–68. https://doi.org/10.1016/j.phytochem.2015.07.012.

124. Ghasemzadeh A, Karbalaii MT, Jaafar HZE, Rahmat A. Phytochemical constituents, antioxidant activity, and antiproliferative properties of black, red, and brown rice bran. Chem Cent J. 2018;12:17. https://doi.org/10.1186/s13065-018-0382-9.
125. Michalak M, Pierzak M, Kręcisz B, Suliga E. Bioactive compounds for skin health: a review. Nutrients. 2021;13:203. https://doi.org/10.3390/nu13010203.
126. Jikah AN, Edo GI. Mechanisms of action by sulphur compounds in Allium sativum. A review. Pharmacol Res Mod Chin Med. 2023;9:100323. https://doi.org/10.1016/j.prmcm.2023.100323.
127. Edo GI, Onoharigho FO, Jikah AN, et al. Cyperus esculentus (tiger nut): an insight into its bioactive compounds, biological activities, nutritional and health benefits. Food Chem Adv. 2023;3: 100511. https://doi.org/10.1016/j.focha.2023.100511.
128. Edo GI, Jikah AN, Onoharigho FO, et al. The ameliorative effects of Vernonia amygdalina extract on superoxide dismutase and glutathione s-transferase on alloxan induced diabetes on male Wistar rats. Food Chem Adv. 2024;4: 100620. https://doi.org/10.1016/j.focha.2024.100620.
129. Edo GI, Ugbune U, Akpoghelie PO, Owheruo JO. Evaluation of physicochemical, phytochemical, anti-bacterial and antioxidant potential of kola nut (cola acuminata): an approach in food, health and nutritional benefits. Vegetos. 2023. https://doi.org/10.1007/s42535-023-00715-0.
130. Anh NH, Kim SJ, Long NP, et al. Ginger on human health: a comprehensive systematic review of 109 randomized controlled trials. Nutrients. 2020;12:157. https://doi.org/10.3390/nu12010157.

131. Edo GI, Onoharigho FO, Jikah AN, et al. Evaluation of the physicochemical, phytochemical and anti-bacterial potential of Zingiber officinale (ginger). Food Chem Adv. 2024;4: 100625. https://doi.org/10.1016/j.focha.2024.100625.

132. Kumavath R, Paul S, Pavithran H, et al. Emergence of cardiac glycosides as potential drugs: current and future scope for cancer therapeutics. Biomolecules. 2021;11:1275. https://doi.org/10.3390/biom11091275.

133. Nikkhah Bodagh M, Maleki I, Hekmatdoost A. Ginger in gastrointestinal disorders: a systematic review of clinical trials. Food Sci Nutr. 2019;7:96–108. https://doi.org/10.1002/fsn3.807.

134. Ku Y-S, Contador CA, Ng M-S, et al. The effects of domestication on secondary metabolite composition in legumes. Front Genet. 2020. https://doi.org/10.3389/fgene.2020.581357.

135. Shah A, Smith DL. Flavonoids in agriculture: chemistry and roles in, biotic and abiotic stress responses, and microbial associations. Agronomy. 2020;10:1209. https://doi.org/10.3390/agronomy10081209.

136. Jafarzadeh A, Jafarzadeh S, Nemati M. Therapeutic potential of ginger against COVID-19: is there enough evidence? J Tradit Chinese Med Sci. 2021;8:267–79. https://doi.org/10.1016/j.jtcms.2021.10.001.

137. Edo GI. Coordination of bioactive phytochemicals from Aloe vera extracts to metal ions; investigation of the metal complexes and bioactive compound formed. Biometals. 2024. https://doi.org/10.1007/s10534-024-00611-3.

138. Ullah A, Munir S, Badshah SL, et al. Important flavonoids and their role as a therapeutic agent. Molecules. 2020;25:5243. https://doi.org/10.3390/molecules25225243.

139. Akpoghelie PO, Edo GI, Ali SI, et al. Effect of processing on the microbiological, proximate, antinutritional and mineral profile of selected yellow cassava varieties and sorghum malt as potential raw materials for alcoholic beverage production. Beverage Plant Res. 2024. https://doi.org/10.48130/bpr-0024-0022.
140. Ninfali P, Antonelli A, Magnani M, Scarpa ES. Antiviral properties of flavonoids and delivery strategies. Nutrients. 2020;12:2534. https://doi.org/10.3390/nu12092534.
141. Akpoghelie PO, Edo GI, Kasar KA, et al. Impact of different nitrogen sources, initial pH and varying inoculum size on the fermentation potential of Saccharomyces cerevisiae on wort obtained from sorghum substrate. Food Mater Res. 2024. https://doi.org/10.48130/fmr-0024-0012.
142. Jikah AN, Edo GI. Turmeric (Curcuma longa): an insight into its food applications, phytochemistry and pharmacological properties. Vegetos. 2024. https://doi.org/10.1007/s42535-024-01038-4.
143. Jikah AN, Edo GI, Makia RS, et al. A review of the therapeutic potential of sulfur compounds in Allium sativum. Meas Food. 2024;15: 100195. https://doi.org/10.1016/j.meafoo.2024.100195.
144. Edo GI, Onoharigho FO, Kasar KA, et al. Evaluation of the anti-inflammatory potential of zingiber officinale on adjuvant-induced arthritis. Adv Tradit Med. 2024. https://doi.org/10.1007/s13596-024-00779-6.
145. Edo GI, Ndudi W, Makia RS, et al. Nutritional immunological effects and mechanisms of chemical constituents from the homology of medicine and food. Phytochem Rev. 2024. https://doi.org/10.1007/s11101-024-10034-0.

146. Soares S, Brandão E, Guerreiro C, et al. Tannins in food: insights into the molecular perception of astringency and bitter taste. Molecules. 2020;25:2590. https://doi.org/10.3390/molecules25112590.
147. Edo GI, Nwachukwu SC, Ali ABM, et al. A review on the composition, extraction and applications of phenolic compounds. Ecol Front. 2024. https://doi.org/10.1016/j.ecofro.2024.09.008.
148. Liu X, Xi K, Wang Y, et al. Evaluation of the contact toxicity and physiological mechanisms of ginger (Zingiber officinale) shoot extract and selected major constituent compounds against Melanaphis sorghi theobald. Horticulturae. 2022;8:944. https://doi.org/10.3390/horticulturae8100944.
149. Yang Z, Wang H, Ying G, et al. Relationship of mycotoxins accumulation and bioactive components variation in ginger after fungal inoculation. Front Pharmacol. 2017. https://doi.org/10.3389/fphar.2017.00331.
150. Demonsais L, Utz-Pugin A, Loubéry S, Lopez-Molina L. Identification of tannic cell walls at the outer surface of the endosperm upon Arabidopsis seed coat rupture. Plant J. 2020;104:567–80. https://doi.org/10.1111/tpj.14994.
151. Edo GI, Nwachukwu SC, Makia RS, et al. Unveiling the Chinese or red date (Ziziphus jujuba); its phytochemical, botanical, industrial and pharmacological properties: a review. Phytochem Rev. 2024. https://doi.org/10.1007/s11101-024-10037-x.
152. Parham S, Kharazi AZ, Bakhsheshi-Rad HR, et al. Antioxidant, antimicrobial and antiviral properties of herbal materials. Antioxidants. 2020;9:1309. https://doi.org/10.3390/antiox9121309.
153. Li H, Rafie R, Xu Z, Siddiqui RA. Phytochemical profile and anti-oxidation activity changes during ginger (Zingiber officinale) harvest: baby ginger

attenuates lipid accumulation and ameliorates glucose uptake in HepG2 cells. Food Sci Nutr. 2022;10:133–44. https://doi.org/10.1002/fsn3.2654.

154. Owheruo JO, Edo GI, Makia RS, et al. Nutritional qualities of cookies made from wheat/cashew nut composite flour. Food Humanit. 2024;3: 100452. https://doi.org/10.1016/j.foohum.2024.100452.

155. Choi J, Lee J, Kim K, et al. Effects of ginger intake on chemotherapy-induced nausea and vomiting: a systematic review of randomized clinical trials. Nutrients. 2022;14:4982. https://doi.org/10.3390/nu14234982.

156. Gupta K, Walton R, Kataria SP. Chemotherapy-induced nausea and vomiting: pathogenesis, recommendations, and new trends. Cancer Treat Res Commun. 2021;26: 100278. https://doi.org/10.1016/j.ctarc.2020.100278.

157. Alharbi KS, Nadeem MS, Afzal O, et al. Gingerol, a natural antioxidant, attenuates hyperglycemia and downstream complications. Metabolites. 2022;12:1274. https://doi.org/10.3390/metabo12121274.

158. Emakpor OL, Edo GI, Jikah AN, et al. Mulching materials effect on soil temperature, moisture content, plant growth and yield of amaranthus plant. Vegetos. 2024. https://doi.org/10.1007/s42535-024-01054-4.

159. Moses RJ, Edo GI, Jikah AN, et al. Cassava consumption and the risk from cyanide poisoning. Vegetos. 2024. https://doi.org/10.1007/s42535-024-01121-w.

160. Alsahli MA, Almatroodi SA, Almatroudi A, et al. 6-Gingerol, a major ingredient of ginger attenuates diethylnitrosamine-induced liver injury in rats through the modulation of oxidative stress and anti-inflammatory activity. Mediators Inflamm. 2021;2021:1–17. https://doi.org/10.1155/2021/6661937.

161. Xi K-Y, Xiong S-J, Li G, et al. Antifungal activity of ginger rhizome extract against Fusarium solani. Horticulturae. 2022;8:983. https://doi.org/10.3390/horticulturae8110983.
162. Ahmed N, Karobari MI, Yousaf A, et al. The antimicrobial efficacy against selective oral microbes, antioxidant activity and preliminary phytochemical screening of zingiber officinale. Infect Drug Resist. 2022;15:2773–85. https://doi.org/10.2147/IDR.S364175.
163. de Nunes CR, Barreto Arantes M, de Menezes Faria Pereira S, et al. Plants as sources of anti-inflammatory agents. Molecules. 2020;25:3726. https://doi.org/10.3390/molecules25163726.
164. Kostelecka K, Bryliński Ł, Komar O, et al. An overview of the spices used for the prevention and potential treatment of gastric cancer. Cancers. 2024;16:1611. https://doi.org/10.3390/cancers16081611.
165. Susanto A, Hartajanie L, Wu C-C. α-Phellandrene enhances the apoptosis of HT-29 cells induced by 5-fluorouracil by modulating the mitochondria-dependent pathway. Oncol Rep. 2024;51:61. https://doi.org/10.3892/or.2024.8720.
166. Saberi F, Sadat Z, Abedzadeh-Kalahroudi M, Taebi M (2014) Effect of Ginger on Relieving Nausea and Vomiting in Pregnancy: A Randomized, Placebo-Controlled Trial. Nurs Midwifery Stud. https://doi.org/10.17795/nmsjournal11841
167. Crichton M, Davidson AR, Innerarity C, et al. Orally consumed ginger and human health: an umbrella review. Am J Clin Nutr. 2022;115:1511–27. https://doi.org/10.1093/ajcn/nqac035.

168. Ghayur MN, Gilani AH. Ginger lowers blood pressure through blockade of voltage-dependent calcium channels. J Cardiovasc Pharmacol. 2005;45:74–80. https://doi.org/10.1097/00005344-200501000-00013.
169. Cerdá B, Marhuenda J, Arcusa R, et al. Ginger in the Prevention of Cardiovascular Diseases. In: Current Topics in Functional Food. IntechOpen. 2022.
170. Arcusa R, Villaño D, Marhuenda J, et al. Potential role of ginger (Zingiber officinale Roscoe) in the prevention of neurodegenerative diseases. Front Nutr. 2022. https://doi.org/10.3389/fnut.2022.809621.
171. Hassan F, Edo GI, Nwosu LC, et al. An inventory of medicinal plants used as sedative, analgesic and blood tonic in Abeokuta, Ogun State, Nigeria. Acta Ecol Sin. 2021; https://doi.org/10.1016/j.chnaes.2021.11.003.
172. Randolph TR, Le A, DeMond J. A modified sodium metabisulfite method to distinguish sickle cell disease from sickle cell trait for use in underdeveloped countries. Am Soc Clin Lab Sci. 2019;32:93–93. https://doi.org/10.29074/ascls.2019002030.
173. Powell-Wiley TM, Poirier P, Burke LE, et al. Obesity and cardiovascular disease: a scientific statement from the american heart association. Circulation. 2021. https://doi.org/10.1161/CIR.0000000000000973.
174. Seo SH, Fang F, Kang I. Ginger (Zingiber officinale) attenuates obesity and adipose tissue remodeling in high-fat diet-fed C57BL/6 mice. Int J Environ Res Public Health. 2021;18:631. https://doi.org/10.3390/ijerph18020631.
175. Suk S, Kwon GT, Lee E, et al. Gingerenone A, a polyphenol present in ginger, suppresses obesity and adipose tissue inflammation in high-fat diet-fed mice. Mol Nutr Food Res. 2017;61:1700139. https://doi.org/10.1002/mnfr.201700139.

176. Rahimlou M, Yari Z, Rayyani E, et al. Effects of ginger supplementation on anthropometric, glycemic and metabolic parameters in subjects with metabolic syndrome: a randomized, double-blind, placebo-controlled study. J Diabetes Metab Disord. 2019;18:119–25. https://doi.org/10.1007/s40200-019-00397-z.
177. Ji E, Jung MY, Park JH, et al. Inhibition of adipogenesis in 3T3-L1 cells and suppression of abdominal fat accumulation in high-fat diet-feeding C57BL/6J mice after downregulation of hyaluronic acid. Int J Obes. 2014;38:1035–43. https://doi.org/10.1038/ijo.2013.202.
178. Jafarnejad S, Keshavarz SA, Mahbubi S, et al. Effect of ginger (Zingiber officinale) on blood glucose and lipid concentrations in diabetic and hyperlipidemic subjects: a meta-analysis of randomized controlled trials. J Funct Foods. 2017;29:127–34. https://doi.org/10.1016/j.jff.2016.12.006.
179. McMillin SL, Evans PL, Taylor WM, et al. Muscle-specific ablation of glucose transporter 1 (GLUT1) does not impair basal or overload-stimulated skeletal muscle glucose uptake. Biomolecules. 2022;12:1734. https://doi.org/10.3390/biom12121734.
180. Hajimoosayi F, Jahanian Sadatmahalleh S, Kazemnejad A, Pirjani R. Effect of ginger on the blood glucose level of women with gestational diabetes mellitus (GDM) with impaired glucose tolerance test (GTT): a randomized double-blind placebo-controlled trial. BMC Complement Med Ther. 2020;20:116. https://doi.org/10.1186/s12906-020-02908-5.
181. Bekkouch O, Dalli M, Harnafi M, et al. Ginger (Zingiber officinale Roscoe), Lemon (Citrus limon L.) juices as preventive agents from chronic liver damage induced by CCl4: a biochemical and histological study. Antioxidants. 2022;11:390. https://doi.org/10.3390/antiox11020390.

182. Shahrajabian MH, Sun W, Cheng Q. Pharmacological uses and health benefits of ginger (Zingiber officinale) in traditional Asian and ancient Chinese medicine, and modern practice. Not Sci Biol. 2019;11:309–19.
183. Shin J-K, Park JH, Kim KS, et al. Antiulcer activity of steamed ginger extract against ethanol/HCl-induced gastric mucosal injury in rats. Molecules. 2020;25:4663. https://doi.org/10.3390/molecules25204663.
184. Mohd Sahardi NFN, Makpol S. Ginger (Zingiber officinale Roscoe) in the prevention of ageing and degenerative diseases: review of current evidence. Evidence-Based Complement Altern Med. 2019;2019:1–13. https://doi.org/10.1155/2019/5054395.
185. Gebashe FC, Naidoo D, Amoo SO, Masondo NA. Cosmeceuticals: a newly expanding industry in South Africa. Cosmetics. 2022;9:77. https://doi.org/10.3390/cosmetics9040077.
186. Al-Atif H. Collagen supplements for aging and wrinkles: a paradigm shift in the field of dermatology and cosmetics. Dermatol Pract Concept. 2022. https://doi.org/10.5826/dpc.1201a18.
187. Esther AdeyeOluwa T (2023) Essential Oil of Ginger: Effect of Cultivation and Uses. In: Ginger—Cultivation and Use. IntechOpen
188. Morgan JP. Jamaica ginger paralysis. Arch Neurol. 1978;35:530. https://doi.org/10.1001/archneur.1978.00500320050011.
189. Menon V, Elgharib M, El-awady R, Saleh E. Ginger: from serving table to salient therapy. Food Biosci. 2021;41: 100934. https://doi.org/10.1016/j.fbio.2021.100934.
190. Szymczak J, Grygiel-Górniak B, Cielecka-Piontek J. Zingiber officinale roscoe: the antiarthritic potential of a popular spice—preclinical and clinical evidence. Nutrients. 2024;16:741. https://doi.org/10.3390/nu16050741.

191. Hend T. Ginger extract attenuates labetalol induced apoptosis, DNA damage, histological and ultrastructural changes in the heart of rat fetuses. Saudi J Biol Sci. 2021;28:440–7. https://doi.org/10.1016/j.sjbs.2020.10.027.

192. Stanisiere J, Mousset P-Y, Lafay S. How safe is ginger rhizome for decreasing nausea and vomiting in women during early pregnancy? Foods. 2018;7:50. https://doi.org/10.3390/foods7040050.

193. Ballester P, Cerdá B, Arcusa R, et al. Effect of ginger on inflammatory diseases. Molecules. 2022;27:7223. https://doi.org/10.3390/molecules27217223.

194. Salem HM, Saad AM, Soliman SM, et al. Ameliorative avian gut environment and bird productivity through the application of safe antibiotics alternatives: a comprehensive review. Poult Sci. 2023. https://doi.org/10.1016/j.psj.2023.102840.

195. Ali MY, Sina AAI, Khandker SS, et al. Nutritional composition and bioactive compounds in tomatoes and their impact on human health and disease: a review. Foods. 2020;10:45. https://doi.org/10.3390/foods10010045.

196. Rupasinghe V, Gunathilake K. Recent perspectives on the medicinal potential of ginger. Bot Targets Ther. 2015. https://doi.org/10.2147/BTAT.S68099.

197. da Fonsêca DV, da Silva Maia Bezerra Filho C, Lima TC, et al. Anticonvulsant essential oils and their relationship with oxidative stress in epilepsy. Biomolecules. 2019;9:835. https://doi.org/10.3390/biom9120835.

198. Ghasemzadeh A, Jaafar HZE, Rahmat A. Synthesis of phenolics and flavonoids in ginger (Zingiber officinale Roscoe) and their effects on

photosynthesis rate. Int J Mol Sci. 2010;11:4539–55. https://doi.org/10.3390/ijms11114539.

199. Imran M., Ghorat F., Ul-Haq I., Ur-Rehman H., Aslam F., Heydari M., Shariati M.A., Okuskhanova E., Yessimbekov Z., Thiruvengadam M., et al. Lycopene as a Natural Antioxidant Used to Prevent Human Health Disorders. Antioxidants. 2020;9:706. doi: 10.3390/antiox9080706.

200. Przybylska S. Lycopene—A bioactive carotenoid offering multiple health benefits: A review. Int. J. Food Sci. Tech. 2019;55:11–32. doi: 10.1111/ijfs.14260.

201. Aziz E., Batool R., Akhtar W., Rehman S., Shahzad T., Malik A., Shariati M.A., Laishevtcev A., Plygun S., Heydari M., et al. Xanthophyll: Health benefits and therapeutic insights. Life Sci. 2020;240:117104. doi: 10.1016/j.lfs.2019.117104.

202. Sara Sara G.Y., Dauda S., Emmanuel A., Bhutto Y.Y., Joseph I. Phytochemical screening and antimicrobial activity of leaf and stem-bark aqueous extracts of Diospyros mespiliformis. Int. J. Biochem. Res. Rev. 2018;22:1–8. doi: 10.9734/IJBCRR/2018/40959.

203. Jiao Y., Reuss L., Wang Y. β-Cryptoxanthin: Chemistry, occurrence, and potential health benefits. Curr. Pharmacol. Rep. 2019;5:20–34. doi: 10.1007/s40495-019-00168-7.

204. Furukawa H. Cultivation technology for vegetable and herb production. In: Anpo M., Fukuda H., Wada T., editors. Plant Factory Using Artificial Light: Adapting to Environmental Disruption and Clues to Agricultural Innovation. Elsevier; Amsterdam, The Netherlands: 2019. pp. 15–23.

205. Wang X., Ma Y., Xu Q., Shikov A.N., Pozharitskaya O.N., Flisyuk E.V., Liu M., Li H., Duez P. Flavonoids and saponins: What have we got or

missed? Phytomedicine. 2023;109:154580. doi: 10.1016/j.phymed.2022.154580.

206. Bonetti F., Brombo G., Zuliani G. Nootropics, functional foods, and dietary patterns for prevention of cognitive decline. In: Watson R.R., editor. Nutrition and Functional Foods for Healthy Aging. Academic Press; Cambridge, MA, USA: 2017. pp. 211–232.

207. Guan L., Fan P., Li S.H., Liang Z., Wu B.H. Inheritance patterns of anthocyanins in berry skin and flesh of the interspecific population derived from teinturier grape. Euphytica. 2019;215:1–14. doi: 10.1007/s10681-019-2342-4.

208. Tsao R. Chemistry and biochemistry of dietary polyphenols. Nutrients. 2010;2:1231–1246. doi: 10.3390/nu2121231.

209. Shahbazi Y., Shavisi N. Limonene. In: Mushtaq M., Farooq A., editors. A Centum of Valuable Plant Bioactives. Academic Press; Cambridge, MA, USA: 2021. pp. 77–91.

210. Eddin L.B., Jha N.K., Meeran M., Kesari K.K., Beiram R., Ojha S. Neuroprotective potential of limonene and limonene containing natural products. Molecules. 2021;26:4535. doi: 10.3390/molecules26154535.

211. Richter G., Hazzah T., Hartsel J.A., Eades J., Hickory B., Makriyannis A. Nutraceuticals. Academic Press; Cambridge, MA, USA: 2021. Cannabis sativa: An overview; pp. 603–624.

212. Cox-Georgian D., Ramadoss N., Dona C., Basu C. Therapeutic and medicinal uses of terpenes. In: Joshee N., Dhekney S., Parajuli P., editors. Medicinal Plants. Springer; Cham, Germany: 2019. pp. 333–359.

213. Hu D., Gao H., Yao X. Biosynthesis of Triterpenoid Natural Products. In: Liu H.-W., Begley T.P., editors. Comprehensive Natural Products III. Elsevier; New York, NY, USA: 2020. pp. 577–612.

214. Morgia G., Privitera S. Phytotherapy in benign prostatic hyperplasia. In: Moriga G., Russo G.I., editors. Lower Urinary Tract Symptoms and Benign Prostatic Hyperplasia. Academic Press; Cambridge, MA, USA: 2018. pp. 135–175.

215. Ashraf R., Bhatti H.N. Stigmasterol. In: Mushtaq M., Anwar F., editors. A Centum of Valuable Plant Bioactives. Academic Press; Cambridge, MA, USA: 2021. pp. 213–232.

216. Lafont R., Dauphin-Villemant C., Warren J.T., Rees H.H. Ecdysteroid chemistry and biochemistry. Ref. Mod. Life Sci. 2005;3:125–195. doi: 10.1016/b978-0-12-809633-8.04026-7.

217. González-Romero J., Guerra-Hernández E.J., Rodríguez-Pérez C. Bioactive compounds from Moringa oleifera as promising protectors of in vivo inflammation and oxidative stress processes. In: Hernandez-Ledesma B., Martinez-Villaluenga C., editors. Current Advances for Development of Functional Foods Modulating Inflammation and Oxidative Stress. Academic Pres; Cambridge, MA, USA: 2022. pp. 379–399.

218. Glencross B. Aquafeed Formulation. Academic Pres; Cambridge, MA, USA: 2016. Understanding the nutritional and biological constraints of ingredients to optimize their application in aquaculture feeds; pp. 33–73.

219. Akihisa T., Zhang J., Manosroi A., Kikuchi T., Manosroi J., Abe M. Limonoids and other secondary metabolites of Azadirachta indica (neem) and Azadirachta indica var. siamensis (Siamese neem), and their

bioactivities. Bioact. Nat. Prod. 2021;68:29–65. doi: 10.1016/b978-0-12-819485-0.00013-x.
220. Sandeep, Ghosh S. Triterpenoids: Structural diversity, biosynthetic pathway, and bioactivity. Bioact. Nat. Prod. 2020;67:411–461. doi: 10.1016/b978-0-12-819483-6.00012-6.
221. Gidley M.J., Yakubov G.E. Functional categorisation of dietary fibre in foods: Beyond "soluble" vs "insoluble". Trends Food Sci. Technol. 2019;86:563–568. doi: 10.1016/j.tifs.2018.12.006.
222. Barber T.M., Kabisch S., Pfeiffer A.F.H., Weickert M.O. The health benefits of dietary fibre. Nutrients. 2020;12:3209. doi: 10.3390/nu12103209.
223. Erkaya T., Dağdemir E., Şengül M. Influence of Cape gooseberry (Physalis peruviana L.) addition on the chemical and sensory characteristics and mineral concentrations of ice cream. Food Res. Int. 2012;45:331–335. doi: 10.1016/j.foodres.2011.09.013.
224. Yalınkılıç B., Kaban G., Kaya M. The effects of different levels of orange fiber and fat on microbiological, physical, chemical and sensorial properties of sucuk. Food Microbiol. 2012;29:255–259. doi: 10.1016/j.fm.2011.07.013.
225. Oz F., Kızıl M., Zaman A., Turhan S. The effects of direct addition of low and medium molecular weight chitosan on the formation of heterocyclic aromatic amines in beef chop. LWT -Food Sci. Technol. 2016;65:861–867. doi: 10.1016/j.lwt.2015.09.023.
226. Oz F., Zaman A., Kaya M. Effect of Chitosan on the Formation of Heterocyclic Aromatic Amines and Some Quality Properties of Meatball. J. Food Process. Preserv. 2017;41:e13065. doi: 10.1111/jfpp.13065.

227. Bedir Y., Karaoğlu M.M. Textural and rheological properties of mulberry leather (pestil) produced with whole grain flours. Int. J. Gastron. Food Sci. 2022;30:100613. doi: 10.1016/j.ijgfs.2022.100613.
228. Azman E.M., Charalampopoulos D., Chatzifragkou A. Acetic acid buffer as extraction medium for free and bound phenolics from dried blackcurrant (Ribes nigrum L.) skins. J. Food Sci. 2020;85:3745–3755. doi: 10.1111/1750-3841.15466.
229. Gopalasatheeskumar K., Parthiban S., Manimaran T., Boopathi T. Phytochemical screening on various extracts (benzene, ethanolic and aqueous) of stem parts of Zanthoxylum rhetsa (roxb.) Dc. Inter.J. Uni. Pharm. Bio Sci. 2017;6:79–91.
230. Laboukhi-Khorsi S., Daoud K., Chemat S. Efficient solvent selection approach for high solubility of active phytochemicals: Application for the extraction of an antimalarial compound from medicinal plants. ACS Sustain. Chem. Eng. 2017;5:4332–4339. doi: 10.1021/acssuschemeng.7b00384.
231. Altemimi A., Lakhssassi N., Baharlouei A., Watson D.G., Lightfoot D.A. Phytochemicals: Extraction, Isolation, and Identification of Bioactive Compounds from Plant Extracts. Plants. 2017;6:42. doi: 10.3390/plants6040042.
232. Banu K.S., Cathrine L. General techniques involved in phytochemical analysis. Int. J. Adv. Res. Chem. Sci. 2015;2:25–32.
233. Scepankova H., Martins M., Estevinho L., Delgadillo I., Saraiva J.A. Enhancement of bioactivity of natural extracts by non-thermal high hydrostatic pressure extraction. Plant Foods Hum. Nut. 2018;73:253–267. doi: 10.1007/s11130-018-0687-9.

234. Bier M.C.J., Medeiros A.B.P., de Oliveira J.S., Côcco L.C., da Luz Costa J., de Carvalho J.C., Soccol C.R. Liquefied gas extraction: A new method for the recovery of terpenoids from agroindustrial and forest wastes. J. Super. Fluids. 2016;110:97–102. doi: 10.1016/j.supflu.2015.12.016.
235. Ivanović M., Islamčević Razboršek M., Kolar M. Innovative extraction techniques using deep eutectic solvents and analytical methods for the isolation and characterization of natural bioactive compounds from plant material. Plants. 2020;9:1428. doi: 10.3390/plants9111428.
236. Mulia K., Putri S., Krisanti E., Nasruddin Natural deep eutectic solvents (NADES) as green solvents for carbon dioxide capture. AIP Conf. Proc. 2017;1923:020022. doi: 10.1063/1.4978095.
237. Paiva A., Craveiro R., Aroso I., Martins M., Reis R.L., Duarte A.R.C. Natural deep eutectic solvents—Solvents for the 21st century. ACS Sustain. Chem. Eng. 2014;2:1063–1071. doi: 10.1021/sc500096j.
238. 135.Hidayat R., Wulandari P. Methods of extraction: Maceration, percolation and decoction. Eureka Herba Indones. 2021;2:73–79. doi: 10.37275/ehi.v2i1.15.
239. Sasikala M., Sundaraganapathy R. Preliminary phytochemical evaluation of hydroalcoholic extract of Ipomoea aquatica Forssk. from Aliyar Riverinein South India. Int. J. Pharma. Bio Sci. 2017;8:356–365. doi: 10.22376/ijpbs.2017.8.3.p356-365.
240. Srivastava P., Bej S., Yordanova K., Wolkenhauer O. Self-attention-based models for the extraction of molecular interactions from biological texts. Biomolecules. 2021;11:1591. doi: 10.3390/biom11111591.
241. Grdiša M., Varga F., Ninčević T., Ptiček B., Dabić D., Biošić M. The extraction efficiency of maceration, UAE and MSPD in the extraction of

pyrethrins from Dalmatian pyrethrum. Agric. Conspec. Sci. 2020;85:257–267.

242. Abegunde S.M., Ayodele-Oduola R.O. Comparison of Efficiency of Different Solvents used for the Extraction of Phytochemicals from the Leaf, Seed and Stem Bark of Calotropis Procera. Int. J. Sci. Res. 2015;4:835–838.

243. Ruiz-Rodríguez A., Palma M., Barroso C.G. Influence of temperature during Pre-fermentative maceration and alcoholic fermentation on the phenolic composition of "Cabernet sauvignon" wines. Foods. 2021;10:1053. doi: 10.3390/foods10051053.

244. Mukherjee P.K. Extraction and other downstream procedures for evaluation of herbal drugs. In: Mukherjee P.K., editor. Quality Control and Evaluation of Herbal Drugs: Evaluating Natural Products and Traditional Medicine. Elsevier; Delhi, India: 2019. pp. 195–236.

245. Chanda S.V., Kaneria M.J. Optimization of conditions for the extraction of antioxidants from leaves of Syzygium cumini L. using different solvents. Food Anal. Methods. 2011;5:332–338. doi: 10.1007/s12161-011-9242-0.

246. Wang Z., Li S., Ge S., Lin S. Review of distribution, extraction methods, and health benefits of bound phenolics in food plants. J. Agric. Food Chem. 2020;68:3330–3343. doi: 10.1021/acs.jafc.9b06574.

247. Zhang Q.W., Lin L.G., Ye W.C. Techniques for extraction and isolation of natural products: A comprehensive review. Chin. Med. 2018;13:1–26. doi: 10.1186/s13020-018-0177-x.

248. Moldovan M.L., Iurian S., Puscas C., Silaghi-Dumitrescu R., Hanganu D., Bogdan C., Vlase L., Oniga I., Benedec D. A design of experiments strategy to enhance the recovery of polyphenolic compounds from Vitis vinifera by-

products through heat reflux extraction. Biomolecules. 2019;9:529. doi: 10.3390/biom9100529.
249. López-Bascón M.A., Luque de Castro M.D. Liquid-Phase Extraction. Elsevier; Amsterdam, The Netherlands: 2020. Soxhlet extraction; pp. 327–354.
250. Shahab M., Roberto S.R., Ahmed S., Colombo R.C., Silvestre J.P., Koyama R., de Souza R.T. Relationship between anthocyanins and skin color of table grapes treated with abscisic acid at different stages of berry ripening. Sci. Hortic. 2020;259:108859. doi: 10.1016/j.scienta.2019.108859.
251. George M.J., Sichilongo K.F., Ramabulana T., Madala N.E., Dubery I.A. Comparison of Soxhlet and reflux techniques for extraction and characterisation of potential endocrine-disrupting compounds from solid waste dumpsite soil. Rnviron. Monit. Assess. 2019;191:149. doi: 10.1007/s10661-019-7294-6.
252. Gopalasatheeskumar K. Significant role of Soxhlet extraction process in phytochemical research. Mintage J. Pharm. Med. Sci. 2018;7:43–47.
253. Patel K., Panchal N., Ingle P. Review of extraction techniques extraction methods: Microwave, ultrasonic, pressurized fluid, soxhlet extraction etc. Int. J. Adv. Res. Chem. Sci. 2019;6:6–21.
254. Alvarez-Rivera G., Bueno M., Ballesteros-Vivas D., Mendiola J.A., Ibañez E. Liquid-Phase Extraction. Elsevier; Amsterdam, The Netherlands: 2020. Pressurized liquid extraction; pp. 375–398.
255. Johnson T.A., Morgan M.V., Aratow N.A., Estee S.A., Sashidhara K.V., Loveridge S.T., Segraves N.L., Crews P. Assessing pressurized liquid extraction for the high-throughput extraction of marine-sponge-derived natural products. J. Nat. Prod. 2010;73:359–364. doi: 10.1021/np900565a.

256. Mustafa A., Turner C. Pressurized liquid extraction as a green approach in food and herbal plants extraction: A review. Anal. Chim. Acta. 2011;703:8–18. doi: 10.1016/j.aca.2011.07.018.
257. Alara O.R., Abdurahman N.H., Ukaegbu C.I. Extraction of phenolic compounds: A review. Curr. Res. Food Sci. 2021;4:200–214. doi: 10.1016/j.crfs.2021.03.011.
258. Plaza M., Turner C. Pressurized hot water extraction of bioactives. Trends Anal. Chem. 2015;71:39–54. doi: 10.1016/j.trac.2015.02.022.
259. Irfan M., Suprajaa P.S., Praveen R., Reddy B.M. Microwave-assisted one-step synthesis of nanohydroxyapetite from fish bones and mussel shells. Mater. Lett. 2021;282:128685. doi: 10.1016/j.matlet.2020.128685.
260. Llompart M., Garcia-Jares C., Celeiro M., Dagnac T. Microwave-assisted extraction. In: Reedijk J., editor. Reference Module in Chemistry, Molecular Sciences and Chemical Engineering. Elsevier; Amsterdam, The Netherlands: 2018. pp. 1–11.
261. Curto S., Taj-Eldin M., Fairchild D., Prakash P. Microwave ablation at 915 MHz vs 2.45 GHz: A theoretical and experimental investigation. Med. Phys. 2015;42:6152–6161. doi: 10.1118/1.4931959.
262. Akhtar I., Javad S., Yousaf Z., Iqbal S., Jabeen K. Review: Microwave assisted extraction of phytochemicals an efficient and modern approach for botanicals and pharmaceuticals. Pakistan J. Pharma. Sci. 2019;32:223–230.
263. Kapoore R., Butler T., Pandhal J., Vaidyanathan S. Microwave-assisted extraction for microalgae: From biofuels to biorefinery. Biology. 2018;7:18. doi: 10.3390/biology7010018.

264. Patil S., Ranveer R.C., Debaje P.P., Kadam J.H., Sahoo A.K. Ultrasound assisted extraction of curcumin. Asian J. Dairy Food Res. 2018;37:250–252. doi: 10.18805/ajdfr.DR-1356.

265. Kumar K., Srivastav S., Sharanagat V.S. Ultrasound assisted extraction (UAE) of bioactive compounds from fruit and vegetable processing by-products: A review. Ultrason. Sonochem. 2021;70:105325. doi: 10.1016/j.ultsonch.2020.105325.

266. Kentish S., Ashokkumar M. The physical and chemical effects of ultrasound. In: Feng H., Barbosa-Canovas G., Weiss J., editors. Technologies for Food and Bioprocessing. Springer; New York, NY, USA: 2010. pp. 1–12.

267. Puri M., Sharma D., Barrow C.J. Enzyme-assisted extraction of bioactives from plants. Trends Biotechnol. 2012;30:37–44. doi: 10.1016/j.tibtech.2011.06.014.

268. Gligor O., Mocan A., Moldovan C., Locatelli M., Crişan G., Ferreira I.C.F.R. Enzyme-assisted extractions of polyphenols—A comprehensive review. Trends Food Sci. Technol. 2019;88:302–315. doi: 10.1016/j.tifs.2019.03.029.

269. Muniglia L., Claisse N., Baudelet P.H., Ricochon G. Enzymatic aqueous extraction (EAE) In: Chemat F., Vian M., editors. Alternative Solvents for Natural Products Extraction. Springer; Berlin/Heidelberg, Germany: 2014. pp. 67–204.

270. Nadar S.S., Rao P., Rathod V.K. Enzyme assisted extraction of biomolecules as an approach to novel extraction technology: A review. Food Res. Int. 2018;108:309–330. doi: 10.1016/j.foodres.2018.03.006.

271. Tabe H., Sukenobe K., Kondo T., Sakurai A., Maruo M., Shimauchi A., Hirano M., Uno S., Kamiya M., Urano Y., et al. Cryogenic fluorescence localization microscopy of spectrally selected individual fret pairs in a water matrix. J. Phys. Chem. B. 2018;122:6906–6911. doi: 10.1021/acs.jpcb.8b03977.
272. Mendiola J.A., Herrero M., Castro-Puyana M., Ibáñez E. Supercritical fluid extraction. In: Rostagno M.A., Prado J.M., editors. Natural Product Extraction Principles and Applications. RSC Publishing; Cambridge, MA, USA: 2013. pp. 196–230.
273. Li R., Xia Z., Li B., Tian Y., Zhang G., Li M., Dong J. Advances in supercritical carbon dioxide extraction of bioactive substances from different parts of Ginkgo biloba L. Molecules. 2021;26:4011. doi: 10.3390/molecules26134011.
274. Majid A., Phull A.R., Khaskheli A.H., Abbasi S., Sirohi M.H., Ahmed I., Ujjan S.H., Jokhio I.A., Ahmed W. Applications and opportunities of supercritical fluid extraction in food processing technologies: A review. Int. J. Adv. Appl. Sci. 2019;6:99–103. doi: 10.21833/ijaas.2019.07.013.
275. Ahmad T., Masoodi F.A., Rather S.A., Wani S.M., Gull A. Supercritical fluid extraction: A review. J. Biol. Chem. Chron. 2019;5:114–122. doi: 10.33980/jbcc.2019.v05i01.019.
276. Geeta H.P., Srinivas G., Champawat P.S. Supercritical Fluid Extraction of Bioactive Compounds from Bioresource: A Review. Int. J. Curr. Microbiol. Appl. Sci. 2020;9:559–566. doi: 10.20546/ijcmas.2020.904.068.
277. Ding X., Liu Q., Hou X., Fang T. Supercritical fluid extraction of metal chelate: A review. Crit. Rev. Anal. Chem. 2017;47:99–118. doi: 10.1080/10408347.2016.1225254.

278. Balasubramaniam V.M., Farkas D., Turek J.E. Preserving Foods through High-Pressure Processing. [(accessed on 1 November 2008)];Food Technol. Mag. 2008 62:32–38. Available online: https://www.ift.org/news-and-publications/food-technology-magazine/issues/2008/november/features/preserving-foods-through-high-pressure-processing.

279. Altuner E.M., Işlek C., Çeter T., Alpas H. High hydrostatic pressure extraction of phenolic compounds from Maclura pomifera fruits. Afr. J. Bio. 2012;11:930–937. doi: 10.1007/s13197-017-2697-2.

280. Purnomo T.A.B., Kurniawan Y.S., Kesuma R.F., Yuliati L. Selection of maceration solvent for natural pigment extraction from red fruit (Pandanus conoideus Lam) Indones. J. Nat. Pigment. 2020;2:8. doi: 10.33479/ijnp.2020.02.1.8.

281. Fernández M.D.L.Á., Boiteux J., Espino M., Gomez F.J.V., Silva M.F. Natural deep eutectic solvents-mediated extractions: The way forward for sustainable analytical developments. Anal. Chim. Acta. 2018;1038:1–10. doi: 10.1016/j.aca.2018.07.059.

282. Costa F.S., Moreira L.S., Silva A.M., Silva R.J., dos Santos M.P., da Silva E.G.P., Grassi M.T., Gonzalez M.H., Amaral C.D. Natural deep eutectic solvent-based microwave-assisted extraction in the medicinal herb sample preparation and elemental determination by ICP OES. J. Food Compos. Anal. 2022;109:104510. doi: 10.1016/j.jfca.2022.104510.

283. Yang Z. Natural deep eutectic solvents and their applications in biotechnology. In: Itoh T., Koo Y.M., editors. Application of Ionic Liquids in Biotechnology. Volume 168. Springer; Cham, Germany: New York, NY, USA: 2018. (Advances in Biochemical Engineering/Biotechnology series).

284. Hikmawanti N., Ramadon D., Jantan I., Mun'im A. Natural deep eutectic solvents (NADES): Phytochemical extraction performance enhancer for pharmaceutical and nutraceutical product development. Plants. 2021;10:2091. doi: 10.3390/plants10102091.

285. Benvenutti L., Zielinski A.A.F., Ferreira S.R.S. Which is the best food emerging solvent: IL, DES or NADES? Trends Food Sci. Technol. 2019;90:133–146. doi: 10.1016/j.tifs.2019.06.003.

286. Erdocia X., Hernández-Ramos F., Morales A., Izaguirre N., de Hoyos-Martínez P.L., Labidi J. Lignin extraction and isolation methods. In: Santos H., Feigueiredo P., editors. Lignin-Based Materials for Biomedical Applications. Elsevier; Amsterdam, The Netherlands: 2021. pp. 61–104.

287. Liu Y., Friesen J.B., McAlpine J.B., Lankin D.C., Chen S.N., Pauli G.F. Natural deep eutectic solvents: Properties, applications, and perspectives. J. Nat. Prod. 2018;81:679–690. doi: 10.1021/acs.jnatprod.7b00945.

288. Yaqoob M., Aggarwal P., Babbar N. Extraction and screening of kinnow (Citrus reticulata L.) peel phytochemicals, grown in Punjab, India. Biomass Convers. Biorefin. 2022;1:1–13. doi: 10.1007/s13399-021-02085-6.

289. Obluchinskaya E.D., Daurtseva A.V., Pozharitskaya O.N., Flisyuk E.V., Shikov A.N. Natural Deep Eutectic Solvents as Alternatives for Extracting Phlorotannins from Brown Algae. Pharma. Chem. J. 2019;53:243–247. doi: 10.1007/s11094-019-01987-0.

290. Sharif M.F., Bennett M.T. The effect of different methods and solvents on the extraction of polyphenols in ginger (Zingiber officinale) J. Teknol. 2016;78:49–54. doi: 10.11113/jt.v78.9943.

291. de Aquino D.S., Roders C., Vessoni A.M., Stevanato N., Da Silva C. Assessment of obtaining sunflower oil from enzymatic aqueous extraction

using protease enzymes. Grasas Aceites. 2022;73:e452. doi: 10.3989/gya.0323211.

292. Hien T.T., Minh N.T. Enhancing the extraction of pumpkin seed (Cucurbita pepo L) for increasing oil yield and its phytosterol content. Food Sci. Appl. Biotechnol. 2021;4:6. doi: 10.30721/fsab2021.v4.i1.104.

293. Jalani N.F. Extraction and purification of phytosterols mixture from palm fatty acid distillate (PFAD) using multistage extraction processes. J. Oil Palm. Res. 2020;33:93–102. doi: 10.21894/jopr.2020.0067.

294. Jafarian Asl P., Niazmand R., Yahyavi F. Extraction of phytosterols and tocopherols from rapeseed oil waste by supercritical CO2 plus co-solvent: A comparison with conventional solvent extraction. Heliyon. 2020;6:e03592. doi: 10.1016/j.heliyon.2020.e03592.

295. Ibrahim N.H., Mahmud M.S., Nurdin S. Microwave-assisted extraction of β-sitosterol from cocoa shell waste. IOP Conf. Ser. Mater. Sci. Eng. 2020;991:012106. doi: 10.1088/1757-899X/991/1/012106.

296. Regalado-Rentería E., Aguirre-Rivera J.R., González-Chávez M.M., Sánchez-Sánchez R., Martínez-Gutiérrez F., Juárez-Flores B.I. Assessment of extraction methods and biological value of seed oil from eight variants of prickly pear fruit (Opuntia spp.) Waste Biomass Valorization. 2018;11:1181–1189. doi: 10.1007/s12649-018-0409-4.

297. Li H., Zhai B., Sun J., Fan Y., Zou J., Cheng J., Zhang X., Shi Y., Guo D. Ultrasound-assisted extraction of total saponins from Aralia taibaiensis: Process optimization, phytochemical characterization, and mechanism of α-glucosidase inhibition. Drug Des. Devel. Ther. 2022;16:83–105. doi: 10.2147/DDDT.S345592.

298. Liu R., Chu X., Su J., Fu X., Kan Q., Wang X., Zhang X. Enzyme-assisted ultrasonic extraction of total flavonoids from Acanthopanax senticosus and their enrichment and antioxidant properties. Processes. 2021;9:1708. doi: 10.3390/pr9101708.
299. Yang G.Y., Song J.N., Chang Y.Q., Wang L., Zheng Y.G., Zhang D., Guo L. Natural deep eutectic solvents for the extraction of bioactive steroidal saponins from Dioscoreae nipponicae rhizoma. Molecules. 2021;26:2079. doi: 10.3390/molecules26072079.
300. Ramli N.H., Yusup S., Quitain A.T., Johari K., Kueh B.W.B. Optimization of saponin extracts using microwave-assisted extraction as a sustainable biopesticide to reduce Pomacea canaliculata population in paddy cultivation. Sustain. Chem. Pharm. 2019;11:23–35. doi: 10.1016/j.scp.2018.12.002.
301. Wu H., Li C., Li Z., Liu R., Zhang A., Xiao Z., Ma L., Li J., Deng S. Simultaneous extraction of oil and tea saponin from Camellia oleifera Abel. seeds under subcritical water conditions. Fuel Process. Technol. 2018;174:88–94. doi: 10.1016/j.fuproc.2018.02.014.
302. Gong X., Zhang Y., Pan J., Qu H. Optimization of the ethanol recycling reflux extraction process for saponins using a design space approach. PLoS ONE. 2014;9:e114300. doi: 10.1371/journal.pone.0114300.
303. Lanjekar K.J., Rathod V.K. Green extraction of glycyrrhizic acid from Glycyrrhiza glabra using choline chloride based natural deep eutectic solvents (NADESs) Process Biochem. 2021;102:22–32. doi: 10.1016/j.procbio.2020.11.023.
304. Shikov A.N., Shikova V.A., Whaley A.O., Burakova M.A., Flisyuk E.V., Whaley A.K., Terninko I.I., Generalova Y.E., Gravel I.V., Pozharitskaya O.N. The Ability of Acid-Based Natural Deep Eutectic Solvents to Co-

Extract Elements from the Roots of Glycyrrhiza glabra L. and Associated Health Risks. Molecules. 2022;27:7690. doi: 10.3390/molecules27227690.
305. Rodrigues V.H., de Melo M.M.R., Portugal I., Silva C.M. Extraction of added-value triterpenoids from Acacia dealbata leaves using supercritical fluid extraction. Processes. 2021;9:1159. doi: 10.3390/pr9071159.
306. Yingngam B., Chiangsom A., Brantner A. Modeling and optimization of microwave-assisted extraction of pentacyclic triterpenes from Centella asiatica leaves using response surface methodology. Ind. Crops. Prod. 2020;147:112231. doi: 10.1016/j.indcrop.2020.112231.
307. Zheng S., Zhang W., Liu S. Optimization of ultrasonic-assisted extraction of polysaccharides and triterpenoids from the medicinal mushroom Ganoderma lucidum and evaluation of their in vitro antioxidant capacities. PLoS ONE. 2020;15:e0244749. doi: 10.1371/journal.pone.0244749.
308. Fernandez-Pastor I., Fernandez-Hernandez A., Perez-Criado S., Rivas F., Martinez A., Garcia-Granados A., Parra A. Microwave-assisted extraction versus Soxhlet extraction to determine triterpene acids in olive skins. J. Sep. Sci. 2017;40:1209–1217. doi: 10.1002/jssc.201601130.
309. Gong T., Liu S., Wang H., Zhang M. Supercritical CO2 fluid extraction, physicochemical properties, antioxidant activities and hypoglycemic activity of polysaccharides derived from fallen Ginkgo leaves. Food Biosci. 2021;42:101153. doi: 10.1016/j.fbio.2021.101153.
310. García P., Fredes C., Cea I., Lozano-Sánchez J., Leyva-Jiménez F.J., Robert P., Vergara C., Jimenez P. Recovery of Bioactive Compounds from Pomegranate (Punica granatum L.) Peel Using Pressurized Liquid Extraction. Foods. 2021;10:203. doi: 10.3390/foods10020203.

311. Hussain S., Sharma M., Bhat R. Valorisation of sea buckthorn pomace by optimization of ultrasonic-assisted extraction of soluble dietary fibre using response surface methodology. Foods. 2021;10:1330. doi: 10.3390/foods10061330.
312. Rivas M.Á., Casquete R., de Guía Córdoba M., Benito M.J., Hernández A., Ruiz-Moyano S., Martín A. Functional properties of extracts and residual dietary fibre from pomegranate (Punica granatum L.) peel obtained with different supercritical fluid conditions. LWT-Food Sc. Tech. 2021;145:111305. doi: 10.1016/j.lwt.2021.111305.
313. Douard L., Bras J., Encinas T., Belgacem M.N. Natural acidic deep eutectic solvent to obtain cellulose nanocrystals using the design of experience approach. Carbohydr. Polym. 2021;252:117136. doi: 10.1016/j.carbpol.2020.117136.
314. Gan J., Huang Z., Yu Q., Peng G., Chen Y., Xie J., Nie S., Xie M. Microwave assisted extraction with three modifications on structural and functional properties of soluble dietary fibers from grapefruit peel. Food Hydrocoll. 2020;101:105549. doi: 10.1016/j.foodhyd.2019.105549.
315. Cheikh Rouhou M., Abdelmoumen S., Thomas S., Attia H., Ghorbel D. Use of green chemistry methods in the extraction of dietary fibers from cactus rackets (Opuntia ficus indica): Structural and microstructural studies. Int. J. Biol. Macromol. 2018;116:901–910. doi: 10.1016/j.ijbiomac.2018.05.090.
316. Gómez A.V., Tadini C.C., Biswas A., Buttrum M., Kim S., Boddu V.M., Cheng H.N. Microwave-assisted extraction of soluble sugars from banana puree with natural deep eutectic solvents (NADES) LWT. 2019;107:79–88. doi: 10.1016/j.lwt.2019.02.052.

317. Liu J., Li Y., Liu W., Qi Q., Hu X., Li S., Lei J., Rong L. Extraction of polysaccharide from Dendrobium nobile Lindl. by subcritical water extraction. ACS Omega. 2019;4:20586–20594. doi: 10.1021/acsomega.9b02550.

318. Kasote DM, Katyare SS, Hegde MV, Bae H (2015) Significance of antioxidant potential of plants and its relevance to therapeutic applications. Int J Biol Sci 11:982

319. Santos HFd, Campos JF, Santos CMd, Balestieri JBP, Silva DB, Carollo CA, Picoli Souza K, Estevinho LM, dos Santos EL (2017) Chemical profile and antioxidant, anti-inflammatory, antimutagenic and antimicrobial activities of geopropolis from the stingless bee *Melipona orbignyi*. Int J Mol Sci 18:953

320. El Toumy S, El Sharabasy F, Ghanem H, El Kady M, Kassem A (2011) Chemical constituents and pharmacological activities of *Zilla spinosa*. Planta Med 77:51

321. Song J, Yeo SG, Hong EH, Lee BR, Kim JW, Kim J, Jeong H, Kwon Y, Kim H, Lee S (2014) Antiviral activity of hederasaponin B from *Hedera helix* against enterovirus 71 subgenotypes C3 and C4a. Biomol Ther 22:41

322. Savithramma N, Rao ML, Suhrulatha D (2011) Screening of medicinal plants for secondary metabolites. Middle East J Sci Res 8:579–584

323. Devkar RA, Chaudhary S, Adepu S, Xavier SK, Chandrashekar KS, Setty MM (2016) Evaluation of antiurolithiatic and antioxidant potential of *Lepidagathis prostrata*: a Pashanbhed plant. Pharm Biol 54:1237–1245

324. Birben E, Sahiner UM, Sackesen C, Erzurum S, Kalayci O (2012) Oxidative stress and antioxidant defense. World Allergy Organ J 5:9

325. Kazeem MI, Ashafa AOT (2016) Antioxidant and inhibitory properties of *Dombeya burgessiae* leaf extracts on enzymes linked to diabetes mellitus. Trans R Soc S Afr 71:167–174

326. Boland DJ, Brooker MIH, Chippendale G, Hall N, Hyland B, Johnston R, Kleinig D, McDonald M, Turner J (2006) Forest trees of Australia. CSIRO publishing, Clayton

327. Cunningham G, Mulham W, Milthorpe P, Leigh J (1992) Plants of western new South Wales. Inkata Press, Sydney

328. Zeid AHA, Farag MA, Hamed MAA, Kandil ZAA, El-Akad RH, El-Rafie HM (2017) Flavonoid chemical composition and antidiabetic potential of *Brachychiton acerifolius* leaves extract. Asian Pac J Trop Biomed 7:389–396

329. Arif N, Yadav V, Singh S, Kushwaha BK, Singh S, Tripathi DK, Vishwakarma K, Sharma S, Dubey N, Chauhan D (2016) Assessment of antioxidant potential of plants in response to heavy metals. In: Singh A, Prasad S, Singh R (eds) Plant responses to xenobiotics. Springer, Berlin, pp 97–125

330. Shah NA, Khan MR, Naz K, Khan MA (2014) Antioxidant potential, DNA protection, and HPLC-DAD analysis of neglected medicinal *Jurinea dolomiaea* roots. BioMed Res Int. https://doi.org/10.1155/2014/726241

331. Sahreen S, Khan MR, Khan RA (2014) Comprehensive assessment of phenolics and antiradical potential of *Rumex hastatus* D. Don. roots. BMC Complement Altern Med 14:47

332. Dhawan D, Gupta J (2017) Comparison of different solvents for phytochemical extraction potential from *Datura metal* plant leaves. Int J Biol Chem 11:17–22

333. Cai Y, Zhang J, Chen NG, Shi Z, Qiu J, He C, Chen M (2016) Recent advances in anticancer activities and drug delivery systems of tannins. Med Res Rev 37:665–701
334. Dzoyem JP, Eloff JN (2015) Anti-inflammatory, anticholinesterase and antioxidant activity of leaf extracts of twelve plants used traditionally to alleviate pain and inflammation in South Africa. J Ethnopharmacol 160:194–201
335. Ng YP, Or TCT, Ip NY (2015) Plant alkaloids as drug leads for Alzheimer's disease. Neurochem Int 89:260–270
336. Hashmi M, Khan A, Farooq U, Khan S (2018) Alkaloids as cyclooxygenase inhibitors in anticancer drug discovery. Curr Protein Pept Sci 19:292–301
337. Chaieb I (2010) Saponins as insecticides: a review. Tunis J Plant Prot 5:39–50
338. Chanda S, Dave R (2009) In vitro models for antioxidant activity evaluation and some medicinal plants possessing antioxidant properties: an overview. Afr J Microbiol Res 3:981–996
339. Alam MN, Bristi NJ, Rafiquzzaman M (2013) Review on in vivo and in vitro methods evaluation of antioxidant activity. Saudi Pharm J 21:143–152
340. Kumaran A (2006) Antioxidant and free radical scavenging activity of an aqueous extract of *Coleus aromaticus*. Food Chem 97:109–114
341. Souza BS, Dantas RF, Cruz A, Sans C, Esplugas S, Dezotti M (2014) Photochemical oxidation of municipal secondary effluents at low H_2O_2 dosage: study of hydroxyl radical scavenging and process performance. Chem Eng J 237:268–276
342. Herraiz T, Galisteo J (2015) Hydroxyl radical reactions and the radical scavenging activity of β-carboline alkaloids. Food Chem 172:640–649

343. Majid M, Khan MR, Shah NA, Haq IU, Farooq MA, Ullah S, Sharif A, Zahra Z, Younis T, Sajid M (2015) Studies on phytochemical, antioxidant, anti-inflammatory and analgesic activities of *Euphorbia dracunculoides*. BMC Complement Altern Med 15:349

344. Wu L, Du Y, Lok J, Lo EH, Xing C (2015) Lipocalin-2 enhances angiogenesis in rat brain endothelial cells via reactive oxygen species and iron-dependent mechanisms. J Neurochem 132:622–628

345. Kanugula AK, Gollavilli PN, Vasamsetti SB, Karnewar S, Gopoju R, Ummanni R, Kotamraju S (2014) Statin-induced inhibition of breast cancer proliferation and invasion involves attenuation of iron transport: intermediacy of nitric oxide and antioxidant defence mechanisms. FEBS J 281:3719–3738

346. Duenas M, Hernandez T, Estrella I (2006) Assessment of in vitro antioxidant capacity of the seed coat and the cotyledon of legumes in relation to their phenolic contents. Food Chem 98:95–103

347. Kilani S, Sghaier MB, Limem I, Bouhlel I, Boubaker J, Bhouri W, Skandrani I, Neffatti A, Ammar RB, Dijoux-Franca MG (2008) In vitro evaluation of antibacterial, antioxidant, cytotoxic and apoptotic activities of the tubers infusion and extracts of *Cyperus rotundus*. Bioresour Technol 99:9004–9008

348. Tan Z, Shahidi F (2013) Antioxidant activity of phytosteryl phenolates in different model systems. Food Chem 138:1220–1224

349. Triantaphyllou GB, Dimitrios Boskou K (2001) Antioxidative properties of water extracts obtained from herbs of the species Lamiaceae. Int J Food Sci Nutr 52:313–317

350. Gupta K, Maurya S, Agarwal S, Kushwaha A, Kumar R (2016) Antioxidant assessment of extracts obtained through hot extraction process. Cell Mol Biol 62:129

351. Jan S, Khan MR, Rashid U, Bokhari J (2013) Assessment of antioxidant potential, total phenolics and flavonoids of different solvent fractions of *Monotheca buxifolia* fruit. Osong Public Health Res Perspect 4:246–254

352. Wang J, Hu S, Nie S, Yu Q, Xie M (2016) Reviews on mechanisms of in vitro antioxidant activity of polysaccharides. Oxid Med Cell Longev. https://doi.org/10.1155/2016/5692852

353. Batool R, Khan MR, Zai JA, Ali S, Maryam S, Naz I, Bibi S (2018) *Brachychiton populneus* (Schott & Endl.) R.Br. ameliorate carbon tetrachloride induced oxidative stress through regulation of endoplasmic reticulum stress markers and inflammatory mediators in Sprague-Dawley male rats. Biomed Pharmacother 107:1601–1610

354. Harborne JB (1998) Phytochemical methods a guide to modern techniques of plant analysis. SSBM, Berlin

355. Trease G, Evans WC (1989) Trease and Evans' pharmacognosy: a physician's Guide to Herbal Medicine, 13th edn. Bailliere Tindall, London, p 912

356. Archana P, Samatha T, Mahitha B, Chamundeswari NR (2012) Preliminary phytochemical screening from leaf and seed extracts of *Senna alata* L. Roxb-an Ethno medicinal plant. Int J Pharm Biol Res 3:82–89

357. Kim DO, Jeong SW, Lee CY (2003) Antioxidant capacity of phenolic phytochemicals from various cultivars of plums. Food Chem 81:321–326

358. Park YS, Jung ST, Kang SG, Heo BG, Arancibia-Avila P, Toledo F, Drzewiecki J, Namiesnik J, Gorinstein S (2008) Antioxidants and proteins in ethylene-treated kiwifruits. Food Chem 107:640–648
359. Van Buren JP, Robinson WB (1969) Formation of complexes between protein and tannic acid. J Agric Food Chem 17:772–777
360. Singh R, Verma PK, Singh G (2012) Total phenolic, flavonoids and tannin contents in different extracts of *Artemisia absinthium*. J Intercult Ethnopharmacol 1:101–104
361. Krishnaiah D, Devi T, Bono A, Sarbatly R (2009) Studies on phytochemical constituents of six Malaysian medicinal plants. J Med Plants Res 3:067–072
362. Obadoni B, Ochuko P (2002) Phytochemical studies and comparative efficacy of the crude extracts of some haemostatic plants in Edo and Delta States of Nigeria. GJPAS 8:203–208
363. Ferguson NM (1956) A Text book of pharmacognosy. New Delhi, MacMilan Company, p 191
364. Halliwell B, Gutteridge JM (1981) Formation of a thiobarbituric-acid-reactive substance from deoxyribose in the presence of iron salts: the role of superoxide and hydroxyl radicals. FEBS Lett 128:347–352
365. Bhaskar H, Balakrishnan N (2009) In vitro antioxidant property of laticiferous plant species from western ghats Tamilnadu, India. Int J Health Res. https://doi.org/10.4314/ijhr.v2i2.55413
366. Dastmalchi K, Dorman HD, Oinonen PP, Darwis Y, Laakso I, Hiltunen R (2008) Chemical composition and in vitro antioxidative activity of a lemon balm (*Melissa officinalis* L.) extract. Food Sci Technol 41:391–400
367. Elzaawely AA, Xuan TD, Koyama H, Tawata S (2007) Antioxidant activity and contents of essential oil and phenolic compounds in flowers and seeds

of *Alpinia zerumbet* (Pers.) BL Burtt. & RM Sm. Food Chem 104:1648–1653

368. Mallet J, Cerrati C, Ucciani E, Gamisans J, Gruber M (1994) Antioxidant activity of plant leaves in relation to their alpha-tocopherol content. Food Chem 49:61–65
369. Landry J, Sutton A, Tafrov ST, Heller RC, Stebbins J, Pillus L, Sternglanz R (2000) The silencing protein SIR2 and its homologs are NAD-dependent protein deacetylases. Proc Natl Acad Sci 97:5807–5811
370. Umamaheswari M, Chatterjee T (2008) In vitro antioxidant activities of the fractions of *Coccinia grandis* L. leaf extract. Afr J Tradit Complement Altern Med 5:61–73
371. Cos, P., Vlietinck, A. J., Berghe, D., Vanden & Maes, L. Anti-infective potential of natural products: how to develop a stronger in vitro 'proof-of-concept'. *J. Ethnopharmacol.* **106**, 290–302. https://doi.org/10.1016/j.jep.2006.04.003 (2006).
372. Um, S., Vang, D., Pin, P. & Chau, D. Trends and determinants of acute respiratory infection symptoms among under-five children in Cambodia: analysis of 2000 to 2014 Cambodia demographic and health surveys. *PLOS Glob. Public Health* **3**, 1–14. https://doi.org/10.1371/journal.pgph.0001440 (2023).
373. Miethke, M. et al. Towards the sustainable discovery and development of new antibiotics. *Nat. Rev. Chem.* **5**, 726–749. https://doi.org/10.1038/s41570-021-00313-1 (2021).
374. Dhingra, S. et al. Microbial resistance movements: an overview of global public health threats posed by antimicrobial resistance, and how best to

counter. *Front. Public Health* **8**, 1–22. https://doi.org/10.3389/fpubh.2020.535668 (2020).

375. Tufa, T. B., Regassa, F., Amenu, K., Stegeman, J. A. & Hogeveen, H. Livestock producers' knowledge, attitude, and behavior (KAB) regarding antimicrobial use in Ethiopia. *Front. Vet. Sci.* **10**, 1–20. https://doi.org/10.3389/fvets.2023.1167847 (2023).
376. Ho, C. S. et al. Antimicrobial resistance: a concise update. *Lancet Microbe* **6** (100947), 1–14. https://doi.org/10.1016/j.lanmic.2024.07.010 (2024).
377. Oliveira, M. et al. An overview of the recent advances in antimicrobial resistance. *Microorganisms* **12**, 1–50. https://doi.org/10.3390/microorganisms12091920 (2024).
378. World Health Organization. Legal status for traditional medicine and complementary/alternative medicine: A worldwide review, 1–189. https://www.who.int/publications/i/item/WHO-EDM-TRM-2001.2 (2001).
379. Fabricant, D. S. & Farnsworth, N. R. The value of plants used in traditional medicine for drug discovery. *Environ. Health Perspect.* **109**, 69–75. https://doi.org/10.1289/ehp.01109s169 (2001).
380. FAO - Food and Agriculture Organization of the United Nations. Non-Wood news 24: an information bulletin on Non-Wood forest products. *Inf. Bull. Non-Wood Prod.* **23**, 1–80. https://www.fao.org/4/i2746e/i2746e00.htm (2011).
381. Kowalska, T. & Sajewicz, M. Thin-layer chromatography (TLC) in the screening of botanicals—its versatile potential and selected

applications. *Molecules* **27** (6607), 1–23. https://doi.org/10.3390/molecules27196607 (2022).

382. Ahmad, I. & Aqil, F. In vitro efficacy of bioactive extracts of 15 medicinal plants against ESβL-producing multidrug-resistant enteric bacteria. *Microbiol. Res.* **162**, 264–275. https://doi.org/10.1016/j.micres.2006.06.010 (2007).

383. Edeoga, H. O., Okwu, D. E. & Mbaebie, B. O. Phytochemical constituents of some Nigerian medicinal plants. *Afr. J. Biotechnol.* **4**, 685–688. https://doi.org/10.5897/AJB2005.000-3127 (2005).

384. Phaniendra, A., Jestadi, D. B. & Periyasamy, L. Free radicals: properties, sources, targets, and their implication in various diseases. *Indian J. Clin. Biochem.* **30**, 11–26. https://doi.org/10.1007/s12291-014-0446-0 (2015).

385. Sharma, T. et al. Phytochemical screening of medicinal plants and study of the effect of phytoconstituents in seed germination. *Tribhuvan Univ. J.* **35**, 1–11. https://doi.org/10.3126/tuj.v35i2.36183 (2020).

386. Paşayeva, L. et al. Optimizing health benefits of walnut (*Juglans regia* L.) agricultural by-products: impact of maceration and Soxhlet extraction methods on phytochemical composition, enzyme Inhibition, antioxidant, antimicrobial, and cytotoxic activities. *Food Biosci.* **64** (105923), 1–23. https://doi.org/10.1016/j.fbio.2025.105923 (2025).

387. Paşayeva, L., Şafak, E. K., Arıgün, T., Fatullayev, H. & Tugay, O. In vitro antioxidant capacity and phytochemical characterization of eryngium kotschyi Boiss. *J. Pharm. Pharmacogn. Res.* **8**, 18–31. https://doi.org/10.56499/jppres19.655_8.1.18 (2020).

388. Rahaman, M. M. et al. Natural antioxidants from some fruits, seeds, foods, natural products, and associated health benefits: an update. *Food Sci. Nutr.* **11**, 1657–1670. https://doi.org/10.1002/fsn3.3217 (2023).

389. Pasayeva, L., Karadeli, H., Ulukus, D., Fatullayev, H. & Tugay, O. Chemical composition and biological activity of the essential oil from eryngium kotschyi Boiss. *J. Essent. Oil Bear. Plants.* **26**, 1055–1066. https://doi.org/10.1080/0972060x.2023.2265959 (2023).

390. Wadood, A. et al. Phytochemical analysis of medicinal plants occurring in local area of Mardan. *Biochem. Anal. Biochem.* **02**, 2–5. https://doi.org/10.4172/2161-1009.1000144 (2013).

391. Hakizamungu, E., van Puyvelde, L., Wéty, M., De Kimpe, N. & Schamp, N. Active principles of tetradenia riparia III. Anti-Trichomonas activity of 8(14), 15-sandaracopimaradiene-7α, 18-diol. *Phyther. Res.* **2**, 207–208. https://doi.org/10.1002/ptr.2650020414 (1988).

392. Baldin, V. P. et al. Anti-mycobacterium tuberculosis activity of essential oil and 6,7-dehydroroyleanone isolated from leaves of tetradenia riparia (Hochst.) Codd (Lamiaceae). *Phytomedicine* **47**, 34–39. https://doi.org/10.1016/j.phymed.2018.04.043 (2018).

393. Van Puyvelde, L. et al. Active principles of tetradenia riparia. I. Antimicrobial activity of 8(14),15-sandaracopimaradiene-7α,18-diol. *J. Ethnopharmacol.* **17**, 269–275. https://doi.org/10.1016/0378-8741(86)90115-7 (1986).

394. Ngbolua, K. et al. Antisickling and antibacterial activities of garcinia punctata Oliv. (Clusiaceae) and tetradenia riparia (Hochst.) Codd (Lamiaceae) from Democratic Republic of the congo. *J. Adv. Med. Life Sci.* **4**, 1–8

(2016). https://www.academia.edu/31378151/Antisickling_and_antibacterial_activities_of_Garcinia_punctata_Oliv_Clusiaceae_and_Tetradenia_riparia_Hochst_Codd_Lamiaceae_from_Democratic_Republic_of_the_Congo
395. Gazim, Z. C. et al. Acaricidal activity of the essential oil from tetradenia riparia (Lamiaceae) on the cattle tick rhipicephalus (Boophilus) Microplus (Acari; Ixodidae). *Exp. Parasitol.* **129**, 175–178. https://doi.org/10.1016/j.exppara.2011.06.011 (2011).
396. Gazim, Z. C. et al. Seasonal variation, chemical composition, and analgesic and antimicrobial activities of the essential oil from leaves of tetradenia riparia (Hochst.) Cdd in Suthern Brazil. *Molecules* **15**, 5509–5524. https://doi.org/10.3390/molecules15085509 (2010).
397. R, M. C. & K, K. N. Assessing the potential of tetradenia riparia in treatment of common skin conditions in rural communities of South Africa. *Afr. J. Microbiol. Res.* **5**, 2942–2945. https://doi.org/10.1016/j.phyplu.2022.100382 (2011).
398. Friedrich, J. C. C. et al. Improved antioxidant activity of a starch and gelatin-based biodegradable coating containing tetradenia riparia extract. *Int. J. Biol. Macromol.* **165**, 1038–1046. https://doi.org/10.1016/j.ijbiomac.2020.09.143 (2020).
399. Da Silva, A. P. S. A. et al. Antimicrobial activity and phytochemical analysis of organic extracts from cleome spinosa Jaqc. *Front. Microbiol.* **7**, 1–10. https://doi.org/10.3389/fmicb.2016.00963 (2016).
400. Ahmed, R. et al. Phenolic contents-based assessment of therapeutic potential of syzygium cumini leaves extract. *PLoS One* **14**, 1–16. https://doi.org/10.1371/journal.pone.0221318 (2019).

401. Olamilosoye, K. P., Akomolafe, R. O., Akinsomisoye, O. S., Adefisayo, M. A. & Alabi, Q. K. The aqueous extract of ocimum gratissimum leaves ameliorates acetic acid-induced colitis via improving antioxidant status and hematological parameters in male Wistar rats. *Egypt. J. Basic Appl. Sci.* **5**, 220–227. https://doi.org/10.1016/j.ejbas.2018.05.006 (2018).

402. Bhattacharya, S., Maity, S., Pramanick, D., Hazra, A. K. & Choudhury, M. HPLC of phenolic compounds, antioxidant and antimicrobial activity of bulbs from three ornithogalum species available in India. *Int. J. Pharm. Pharm. Sci.* **8**, 187–192 (2016). https://www.academia.edu/download/110482462/482240193.pdf

403. Nugraha, S. E., Suryadi, A. & Erly Sitompul. Antibacterial activity of Ethyl acetate fraction of passion fruit Peel (Passiflora Edulis Sims) on Staphylococcus aureus and Escherichia coli. *Indones. J. Pharm. Clin. Res.* **2**, 07–12. https://doi.org/10.32734/idjpcr.v2i1.972 (2019).

404. Wang, C. Y., Chen, Y. W. & Hou, C. Y. Antioxidant and antibacterial activity of seven predominant terpenoids. *Int. J. Food Prop.* **22**, 230–238. https://doi.org/10.1080/10942912.2019.1582541 (2019).

405. Gutiérrez-Del-río, I. et al. Terpenoids and polyphenols as natural antioxidant agents in food preservation. *Antioxidants* **10**, 1–33. https://doi.org/10.3390/antiox10081264 (2021).

406. Zareiyan, F. & Khajehsharifi, H. In-vitro phytochemical analysis of essential oil and methanolic and hydromethanolic extracts of ocimum gratissimum. *J. Plant Biochem. Biotechnol.* **31**, 894–906. https://doi.org/10.1007/s13562-022-00768-3 (2022).

407. Vieira, R. F., Grayer, R. J., Paton, A. & Simon, J. E. Genetic diversity of ocimum gratissimum L. based on volatile oil constituents, flavonoids and

RAPD markers. *Biochem. Syst. Ecol.* **29**, 287–304. https://doi.org/10.1016/S0305-1978(00)00062-4 (2001).

408. Figueroa-Merma, A. et al. Bioactive compounds characterisation of Peruvian dysphania ambrosioides (L.) Mosyakin & clemants leaves by GC/MS and UPLC–ESI–Q/TOF–MSn techniques. *Int. J. Food Sci. Technol.* **58**, 1219–1229. https://doi.org/10.1111/ijfs.16270 (2023).
409. Chikezie, I. O. Determination of minimum inhibitory concentration (MIC) and minimum bactericidal concentration (MBC) using a novel Dilution tube method. *Afr. J. Microbiol. Res.* **11**, 977–980. https://doi.org/10.5897/AJMR2017.8545 (2017).
410. Adil, M. et al. Phytochemical screening, HPLC analysis, antimicrobial and antioxidant effect of euphorbia parviflora L. (Euphorbiaceae Juss). *Sci. Rep.* **14**, 1–10. https://doi.org/10.1038/s41598-024-55905-w (2024).
411. Kumar, S. & Pandey, A. K. Medicinal attributes of solanum xanthocarpum fruit consumed by several tribal communities as food: an in vitro antioxidant, anticancer and anti HIV perspective. *BMC Complement. Altern. Med.* **14**, 1–8. https://doi.org/10.1186/1472-6882-14-112 (2014).
412. Hassanpour, S. H. & Doroudi, A. Review of the antioxidant potential of flavonoids as a subgroup of polyphenols and partial substitute for synthetic antioxidants. *Avicenna J. Phytomed.* **13**, 354–376. https://doi.org/10.22038/ajp.2023.21774 (2023).
413. Pękal, A. & Pyrzynska, K. Evaluation of aluminium complexation reaction for flavonoid content assay. *Food Anal. Methods* **7**, 1776–1782. https://doi.org/10.1007/s12161-014-9814-x (2014).
414. Bag, A. & Chattopadhyay, R. R. Evaluation of synergistic antibacterial and antioxidant efficacy of essential oils of spices and herbs in

combination. *PLoS One* **10**, 1–17. https://doi.org/10.1016/j.indcrop.2020.112569 (2015).

415. Golus, J., Sawicki, R., Widelski, J. & Ginalska, G. The agar microdilution method—a new method for antimicrobial susceptibility testing for essential oils and plant extracts. *J. Appl. Microbiol.* **121**, 1291–1299. https://doi.org/10.1111/jam.13253 (2016).
416. Cicco, N., Lanorte, M. T., Paraggio, M., Viggiano, M. & Lattanzio, V. A reproducible, rapid and inexpensive Folin–Ciocalteu micro-method in determining phenolics of plant methanol extracts. *Microchem. J.* **91**, 107–110. https://doi.org/10.1016/j.microc.2008.08.011 (2009).
417. Okigbo, R.N.; Anuagasi, C.L.; Amadi, J.E. Advances in selected medicinal and aromatic plants indigenous to Africa. *J. Med. Plants Res.* **2009**, *3*, 86–95.
418. Chaachouay, N.; Azeroual, A.; Ansari, M.K.A.; Zidane, L. Use of Plants as Medicines and Aromatics by Indigenous Communities of Morocco: Pharmacognosy, Ecology and Conservation. In *Plants as Medicine and Aromatics*; CRC Press: Boca Raton, FL, USA, 2023; pp. 33–44.
419. Ansari, M.K.A.; Iqbal, M.; Chaachouay, N.; Ansari, A.A.; Owens, G. The Concept and Status of Medicinal and Aromatic Plants: History, Pharmacognosy, Ecology, and Conservation. In *Plants as Medicine and Aromatics*; CRC Press: Boca Raton, FL, USA, 2023; pp. 129–144.
420. Chaachouay, N.; Douira, A.; Hassikou, R.; Brhadda, N.; Dahmani, J.; Belahbib, N.; Ziri, R.; Zidane, L. Etude Floristique et Ethnomédicinale des Plantes Aromatiques et Médicinales dans le Rif (Nord du Maroc). Ph.D. Thesis, Université Ibn Tofail, Kénitra, Morocco, 2020. Available

online: **https://tel.archives-ouvertes.fr/tel-03376377** (accessed on 18 October 2021).

421. Orch, H.; Chaachouay, N.; Douiri, E.M.; Faiz, N.; Zidane, L.; Douira, A. Use of medicinal plants in dermato-cosmetology: An ethnobotanical study among the population of Izarène. *Jordan J. Pharm. Sci.* **2021**, *14*, 323–340.
422. Benkhnigue, O.; Chaachouay, N.; Khamar, H.; El Azzouzi, F.; Douira, A.; Zidane, L. Ethnobotanical and ethnopharmacological study of medicinal plants used in the treatment of anemia in the region of Haouz-Rehamna (Morocco). *J. Pharm. Pharmacogn. Res.* **2022**, *10*, 279–302.
423. Avery, L.M.; Hains, B.J. Oral traditions: A contextual framework for complex science concepts—Laying the foundation for a paradigm of promise in rural science education. *Cult. Stud. Sci. Educ.* **2017**, *12*, 129–166.
424. d'Avigdor, E.; Wohlmuth, H.; Asfaw, Z.; Awas, T. The current status of knowledge of herbal medicine and medicinal plants in Fiche, Ethiopia. *J. Ethnobiol. Ethnomed.* **2014**, *10*, 38.
425. Katiyar, C.; Gupta, A.; Kanjilal, S.; Katiyar, S. Drug discovery from plant sources: An integrated approach. *Ayu* **2012**, *33*, 10.
426. Shakya, A.K. Medicinal plants: Future source of new drugs. *Int. J. Herb. Med.* **2016**, *4*, 59–64.
427. Rates, S.M.K. Plants as source of drugs. *Toxicon* **2001**, *39*, 603–613.
428. Jia, W.; Gao, W.; Yan, Y.; Wang, J.; Xu, Z.; Zheng, W.; Xiao, P. The rediscovery of ancient Chinese herbal formulas. *Phytother. Res.* **2004**, *18*, 681–686.
429. Salim, A.A.; Chin, Y.-W.; Kinghorn, A.D. Drug discovery from plants. In *Bioactive Molecules and Medicinal Plants*; Springer: Berlin/Heidelberg, Germany, 2008; pp. 1–24.

430. Chin, Y.-W.; Balunas, M.J.; Chai, H.B.; Kinghorn, A.D. Drug discovery from natural sources. *AAPS J.* **2006**, *8*, E239–E253.

431. Mohr, C. Plant Made Pharmaceuticals (PMPs) as Medicinal Products for Human Use—A Review of Current Regulatory Issues and Challenges to Achieve a Marketing Authorisation in the EU. 2015. Available online: **https://www.dgra.de/media/pdf/studium/masterthesis/master_mohr_c.pdf** (accessed on 5 November 2015).

432. Subramoniam, A. Present scenario, challenges and future perspectives in plant based medicine development. *Ann. Phytomed* **2014**, *3*, 31–36.

433. Veeresham, C. Natural products derived from plants as a source of drugs. *J. Adv. Pharm. Technol. Res.* **2012**, *3*, 200.

434. Aboelsoud, N.H. Herbal medicine in ancient Egypt. *J. Med. Plants Res.* **2010**, *4*, 82–86.

435. Sam, S. Importance and effectiveness of herbal medicines. *J. Pharmacogn. Phytochem.* **2019**, *8*, 354–357.

436. Yaniv, Z. Introduction: Medicinal Plants in Ancient Traditions. In *Medicinal and Aromatic Plants of the Middle-East*; Yaniv, Z., Dudai, N., Eds.; Medicinal and Aromatic Plants of the World; Springer: Dordrecht, The Netherlands, 2014; Volume 2, pp. 1–7.

437. Sendker, J.; Sheridan, H. History and Current Status of Herbal Medicines. In *Toxicology of Herbal Products*; Pelkonen, O., Duez, P., Vuorela, P.M., Vuorela, H., Eds.; Springer International Publishing: Cham, Switzerland, 2017; pp. 11–277.

438. Msomi, N.Z.; Simelane, M.B. Herbal Medicine. In *Herbal Medicine*; IntechOpen: London, UK, 2018.

439. Forshaw, R. Before Hippocrates. Healing practices in ancient Egypt. In *Medicine, Healing and Performance*; Oxbow Books: Oxford, UK, 2014; pp. 25–41.
440. David, R.; Forshaw, R. *Medicine and Healing Practices in Ancient Egypt*; Liverpool University Press: Liverpool, UK, 2023; Available online: https://books.google.com/books?hl=fr&lr=&id=gbjYEAAAQBAJ&oi=fnd&pg=PR1&dq=Ancient+Egyptian+Healing+Practices+&ots=TEZbQd8Fk6&sig=ZoI0NRKi_KCTGMEx3RuKtHF1Svw (accessed on 8 November 2023).
441. Sze, D.M.; Miller, K.; Neilan, B. Development of taxol and other endophyte produced anti-cancer agents. *Recent Pat. Anticancer Drug Discov.* **2008**, *3*, 14–19.
442. Leeson, P.D.; Springthorpe, B. The influence of drug-like concepts on decision-making in medicinal chemistry. *Nat. Rev. Drug Discov.* **2007**, *6*, 881–890.
443. Pan, S.-Y.; Zhou, S.-F.; Gao, S.-H.; Yu, Z.-L.; Zhang, S.-F.; Tang, M.-K.; Sun, J.-N.; Ma, D.-L.; Han, Y.-F.; Fong, W.-F. New perspectives on how to discover drugs from herbal medicines: CAM's outstanding contribution to modern therapeutics. *Evid.-Based Complement. Alternat. Med.* **2013**, *2013*, 627375.
444. Buhner, S.H. *The Secret Teachings of Plants: The Intelligence of the Heart in the Direct Perception of Nature*; Inner Traditions/Bear & Co.: Rochester, VT, USA, 2004; Available online: **https://books.google.com/books?hl=fr&lr=&id=GgRGF_uDp9AC&oi=fnd&pg=PP1&dq=Indigenous+and+traditional+systems+of+medicine+have+amassed+a+vast+amount+of+infor-**

mation+about+the+medicinal+qualities+of+plants+over+several+generations.+&ots=8-6OGOnw4r&sig=AEKSaerOcKYWhnhep-SMHInx7lc (accessed on 7 November 2023).

445. Grynkiewicz, G.; Gadzikowska, M. Tropane alkaloids as medicinally useful natural products and their synthetic derivatives as new drugs. *Pharmacol. Rep.* **2008**, *60*, 439.

446. Van Agtmael, M.A.; Eggelte, T.A.; Van Boxtel, C.J. Artemisinin drugs in the treatment of malaria: From medicinal herb to registered medication. *Trends Pharmacol. Sci.* **1999**, *20*, 199–205.

447. World Health Organization. *WHO Traditional Medicine Strategy: 2014-2023*; World Health Organization: Geneva, Switzerland, 2013.

448. Lefevere, H.; Bauters, L.; Gheysen, G. Salicylic acid biosynthesis in plants. *Front. Plant Sci.* **2020**, *11*, 338.

449. Patole, J.; Shingnapurkar, D.; Padhye, S.; Ratledge, C. Schiff base conjugates of p-aminosalicylic acid as antimycobacterial agents. *Bioorg. Med. Chem. Lett.* **2006**, *16*, 1514–1517.

450. Zhang, M.; Yang, J.; Cai, Z.; Feng, Y.; Wang, Y.; Zhang, D.; Pan, X. Detection of engineered nanoparticles in aquatic environments: Current status and challenges in enrichment, separation, and analysis. *Environ. Sci. Nano* **2019**, *6*, 709–735.

451. Coley, P.D.; Heller, M.V.; Aizprua, R.; Araúz, B.; Flores, N.; Correa, M.; Gupta, M.; Solis, P.N.; Ortega-Barría, E.; Romero, L.I.; et al. Using ecological criteria to design plant collection strategies for drug discovery. *Front. Ecol. Environ.* **2003**, *1*, 421–428.

452. Maden, K. Plant collection and herbarium techniques. *Our Nat.* **2004**, *2*, 53–57.

453. Altemimi, A.; Lakhssassi, N.; Baharlouei, A.; Watson, D.G.; Lightfoot, D.A. Phytochemicals: Extraction, isolation, and identification of bioactive compounds from plant extracts. *Plants* **2017**, *6*, 42.

454. Vinci, G.; Maddaloni, L.; Prencipe, S.A.; Orlandini, E.; Sambucci, M. Simple and reliable eco-extraction of bioactive compounds from dark chocolate by Deep Eutectic Solvents. A sustainable study. *Int. J. Food Sci. Technol.* **2023**, *58*, 4051–4065.

455. Machado, B.A.S.; Pereira, C.G.; Nunes, S.B.; Padilha, F.F.; Umsza-Guez, M.A. Supercritical Fluid Extraction Using CO_2: Main Applications and Future Perspectives. *Sep. Sci. Technol.* **2013**, *48*, 2741–2760.

456. Sapkale, G.N.; Patil, S.M.; Surwase, U.S.; Bhatbhage, P.K. Supercritical fluid extraction. *Int. J. Chem. Sci.* **2010**, *8*, 729–743.

457. Beaufils, N.; Boucher, J.; Peydecastaing, J.; Rigal, L.; Vilarem, G.; Villette, M.-J.; Candy, L.; Pontalier, P.-Y. The effect of time and temperature on the extraction of xylose and total phenolic compounds with pressurized hot water from hardwood species used for pulp and paper production in the South of France. *Bioresour. Technol. Rep.* **2021**, *16*, 100832.

458. Calvo-Flores, F.G.; Monteagudo-Arrebola, M.J.; Dobado, J.A.; Isac-García, J. Green and Bio-Based Solvents. *Top. Curr. Chem.* **2018**, *376*, 18.

459. Popoola, L.T. Progress on pharmaceutical drugs, plant extracts and ionic liquids as corrosion inhibitors. *Heliyon* **2019**, *5*, e01143. Available online: **https://www.cell.com/heliyon/pdf/S2405-8440(18)33426-1.pdf** (accessed on 18 December 2023).

460. Usmani, Z.; Sharma, M.; Tripathi, M.; Lukk, T.; Karpichev, Y.; Gathergood, N.; Singh, B.N.; Thakur, V.K.; Tabatabaei, M.; Gupta, V.K. Biobased

natural deep eutectic system as versatile solvents: Structure, interaction and advanced applications. *Sci. Total Environ.* **2023**, *881*, 163002.

461. Ghamartale, A.; Afzali, S.; Rezaei, N.; Zendehboudi, S. *Asphaltene Deposition Control by Chemical Inhibitors: Theoretical and Practical Prospects*; Gulf Professional Publishing: Cambridge, MA, USA, 2021.

462. Bochkov, D.V.; Sysolyatin, S.V.; Kalashnikov, A.I.; Surmacheva, I.A. Shikimic acid: Review of its analytical, isolation, and purification techniques from plant and microbial sources. *J. Chem. Biol.* **2012**, *5*, 5–17.

463. Bajpai, V.K.; Majumder, R.; Park, J.G. Isolation and purification of plant secondary metabolites using column-chromatographic technique. *Bangladesh J. Pharmacol.* **2016**, *11*, 844–848.

464. Huang, Y.; Wang, S.; Cai, Q.; Jin, H. Effective methods for isolation and purification of extracellular vesicles from plants. *J. Integr. Plant Biol.* **2021**, *63*, 2020–2030.

465. Araújo, A.S.F.; Monteiro, R.T.R. Plant bioassays to assess toxicity of textile sludge compost. *Sci. Agric.* **2005**, *62*, 286–290.

466. Grant, W.F. The present status of higher plant bioassays for the detection of environmental mutagens. *Mutat. Res. Mol. Mech. Mutagen.* **1994**, *310*, 175–185.

467. Hu, W.; Yu, A.; Wang, S.; Bai, Q.; Tang, H.; Yang, B.; Wang, M.; Kuang, H. Extraction, Purification, Structural Characteristics, Biological Activities, and Applications of the Polysaccharides from *Zingiber officinale* Roscoe. (Ginger): A Review. *Molecules* **2023**, *28*, 3855.

468. Frederick, S.E.; Newcomb, E.H.; Vigil, E.L.; Wergin, W.P. Fine-structural characterization of plant microbodies. *Planta* **1968**, *81*, 229–252.

469. Jin, H.; Geng, Y.; Yu, Z.; Tao, K.; Hou, T. Lead optimization and anti-plant pathogenic fungi activities of daphneolone analogues from Stellera chamaejasme L. *Pestic. Biochem. Physiol.* **2009**, *93*, 133–137.

470. Bregman, H.; Simard, J.R.; Andrews, K.L.; Ayube, S.; Chen, H.; Gunaydin, H.; Guzman-Perez, A.; Hu, J.; Huang, L.; Huang, X.; et al. The Discovery and Hit-to-Lead Optimization of Tricyclic Sulfonamides as Potent and Efficacious Potentiators of Glycine Receptors. *J. Med. Chem.* **2017**, *60*, 1105–1125.

471. Kayser, O. *Medicinal Plant Biotechnology*; Wiley-Vch Verlag GmbH & Co.: Weinheim, Germany, 2007; Available online: **https://ds.amu.edu.et/xmlui/bitstream/handle/123456789/10990/%5Bed._by_Jorg_Knablein%5D_Medicinal_Plant_Biotechnolo.pdf?sequence=1&isAllowed=y** (accessed on 7 November 2023).

472. Puzari, U.; Fernandes, P.A.; Mukherjee, A.K. Pharmacological re-assessment of traditional medicinal plants-derived inhibitors as antidotes against snakebite envenoming: A critical review. *J. Ethnopharmacol.* **2022**, *292*, 115208.

473. DeLong, D.C., Jr. Defining biodiversity. *Wildl. Soc. Bull.* **1996**, *24*, 738–749.

474. Testai, L.; Calderone, V. Nutraceutical value of citrus flavanones and their implications in cardiovascular disease. *Nutrients* **2017**, *9*, 502.

475. Hussain, S.Z.; Naseer, B.; Qadri, T.; Fatima, T.; Bhat, T.A. Peach (Prunus Persica)—Morphology, Taxonomy, Composition and Health Benefits. In *Fruits Grown in Highland Regions of the Himalayas*; Springer: Cham, Switzerland, 2021; pp. 207–217.

476. Yadav, M.; Jain, S.; Bhardwaj, A.; Nagpal, R.; Puniya, M.; Tomar, R.; Singh, V.; Parkash, O.; Prasad, G.B.K.S.; Marotta, F.; et al. Biological and Medicinal Properties of Grapes and Their Bioactive Constituents: An Update. *J. Med. Food* **2009**, *12*, 473–484.
477. Singh, B.N.; Shankar, S.; Srivastava, R.K. Green tea catechin, epigallocatechin-3-gallate (EGCG): Mechanisms, perspectives and clinical applications. *Biochem. Pharmacol.* **2011**, *82*, 1807–1821.
478. Fischer, S.R. *History of Writing*; Reaktion Books: London, UK, 2003.
479. Chaachouay, N.; Douira, A.; Zidane, L. Herbal Medicine Used in the Treatment of Human Diseases in the Rif, Northern Morocco. *Arab. J. Sci. Eng.* **2022**, *47*, 131–153.
480. Chaachouay, N.; Benkhnigue, O.; Fadli, M.; El Ibaoui, H.; El Ayadi, R.; Zidane, L. Ethnobotanical and ethnopharmacological study of medicinal and aromatic plants used in the treatment of respiratory system disorders in the Moroccan Rif. *Ethnobot. Res. Appl.* **2019**, *18*, 1–16.
481. Chaachouay, N.; Azeroual, A.; Douira, A.; Zidane, L. Ethnoveterinary practices of medicinal plants among the Zemmour and Zayane tribes, Middle Atlas, Morocco. *S. Afr. J. Bot.* **2022**, *151*, 826–840.
482. Chaachouay, N.; Azeroual, A.; Bencharki, B.; Douira, A.; Zidane, L. Ethnoveterinary medicines plants for animal therapy in the Rif, North of Morocco. *S. Afr. J. Bot.* **2022**, *147*, 176–191.
483. Houghton, P.J. The role of plants in traditional medicine and current therapy. *J. Altern. Complement. Med.* **1995**, *1*, 131–143.
484. Chaachouay, N.; Benkhnigue, O.; Fadli, M.; El Ayadi, R.; Zidane, L. Ethnobotanical study of medicinal plants used to treat osteoarticular diseases

in the Moroccan Rif, Morocco. *J. Pharm. Pharmacogn. Res.* **2019**, *7*, 454–470.

485. Hosseinzadeh, S.; Jafarikukhdan, A.; Hosseini, A.; Armand, R. The application of medicinal plants in traditional and modern medicine: A review of Thymus vulgaris. *Int. J. Clin. Med.* **2015**, *6*, 635.
486. Karunamoorthi, K.; Jegajeevanram, K.; Vijayalakshmi, J.; Mengistie, E. Traditional medicinal plants: A source of phytotherapeutic modality in resource-constrained health care settings. *J. Evid.-Based Complement. Altern. Med.* **2013**, *18*, 67–74.
487. Sofowora, A.; Ogunbodede, E.; Onayade, A. The role and place of medicinal plants in the strategies for disease prevention. *Afr. J. Tradit. Complement. Altern. Med.* **2013**, *10*, 210–229.
488. Singh, H.; Bharadvaja, N. Treasuring the computational approach in medicinal plant research. *Prog. Biophys. Mol. Biol.* **2021**, *164*, 19–32.
489. Rasoulian, B.; Kheirandish, F. Herbal medicines: From traditional medicine to modern experimental approaches. *Herb. Med. J. Herb. Med. J.* **2017**, *2*, 1–2.
490. Hefferon, K. *Let Thy Food Be Thy Medicine: Plants and Modern Medicine*; OUP USA: New York, NY, USA, 2012; ISBN 978-0-19-987397-5.
491. Jovovic, Z.; Andjelkovic, V.; Przulj, N.; Mandic, D. Untapped Genetic Diversity of Wild Relatives for Crop Improvement. In *Rediscovery of Genetic and Genomic Resources for Future Food Security*; Salgotra, R.K., Zargar, S.M., Eds.; Springer: Singapore, 2020; pp. 25–65.
492. Inoue, M.; Hayashi, S.; Craker, L.E. Role of medicinal and aromatic plants: Past, present, and future. In *Pharmacognosy-Medicinal Plants*; IntechOpen: London, UK, 2019.

493. Mathur, S.; Hoskins, C. Drug development: Lessons from nature. *Biomed. Rep.* **2017**, *6*, 612–614.

494. Abdel-Aziz, S.M.; Aeron, A.; Kahil, T.A. Health Benefits and Possible Risks of Herbal Medicine. In *Microbes in Food and Health*; Garg, N., Abdel-Aziz, S.M., Aeron, A., Eds.; Springer International Publishing: Cham, Switzerland, 2016; pp. 97–116.

495. Valecha, N.; Looareesuwan, S.; Martensson, A.; Mohammed Abdulla, S.; Krudsood, S.; Tangpukdee, N.; Mohanty, S.; Mishra, S.K.; Tyagi, P.K.; Sharma, S.K. Arterolane, a new synthetic trioxolane for treatment of uncomplicated Plasmodium falciparum malaria: A phase II, multicenter, randomized, dose-finding clinical trial. *Clin. Infect. Dis.* **2010**, *51*, 684–691.

496. Salam, A.M.; Quave, C.L. Opportunities for plant natural products in infection control. *Curr. Opin. Microbiol.* **2018**, *45*, 189–194.

497. Chaachouay, N.; Douira, A.; Zidane, L. COVID-19, prevention and treatment with herbal medicine in the herbal markets of Salé Prefecture, North-Western Morocco. *Eur. J. Integr. Med.* **2021**, *42*, 101285.

498. Lahlou, M. The success of natural products in drug discovery. *Pharmacol. Pharm.* **2013**, *4*, 17–31.

499. Pascolutti, M.; Quinn, R.J. Natural products as lead structures: Chemical transformations to create lead-like libraries. *Drug Discov. Today* **2014**, *19*, 215–221.

500. Böttcher, C.; Harvey, K.; Forde, C.G.; Boss, P.K.; Davies, C. Auxin treatment of pre-veraison grape (Vitis vinifera L.) berries both delays ripening and increases the synchronicity of sugar accumulation. *Aust. J. Grape Wine Res.* **2011**, *17*, 1–8.

501. Majolo, F.; Delwing, L.K.D.O.B.; Marmitt, D.J.; Bustamante-Filho, I.C.; Goettert, M.I. Medicinal plants and bioactive natural compounds for cancer treatment: Important advances for drug discovery. *Phytochem. Lett.* **2019**, *31*, 196–207.
502. Cassano, T.; Villani, R.; Pace, L.; Carbone, A.; Bukke, V.N.; Orkisz, S.; Avolio, C.; Serviddio, G. From Cannabis sativa to cannabidiol: Promising therapeutic candidate for the treatment of neurodegenerative diseases. *Front. Pharmacol.* **2020**, *11*, 124.
503. Chaachouay, N.; Azeroual, A.; Bencharki, B.; Douira, A.; Zidane, L. *Cannabis sativa* L.: A Review on Traditional Uses, Botany, Phytochemistry, and Pharmacological Aspects. *Tradit. Integr. Med.* **2023**, *8*, 97–116.
504. Wijeweera, G.; Wijekoon, N.; Gonawala, L.; Imran, Y.; Mohan, C.; De Silva, K.R.D. Therapeutic Implications of Some Natural Products for Neuroimmune Diseases: A Narrative of Clinical Studies Review. *Evid.-Based Complement. Alternat. Med.* **2023**, *2023*, 5583996.
505. Khan, M.S.A.; Ahmad, I. Herbal medicine: Current trends and future prospects. In *New Look to Phytomedicine*; Elsevier: Amsterdam, The Netherlands, 2019; pp. 3–13.
506. Thomford, N.E.; Senthebane, D.A.; Rowe, A.; Munro, D.; Seele, P.; Maroyi, A.; Dzobo, K. Natural products for drug discovery in the 21st century: Innovations for novel drug discovery. *Int. J. Mol. Sci.* **2018**, *19*, 1578.
507. Cragg, G.M.; Newman, D.J. Natural product drug discovery in the next millennium. *Pharm. Biol.* **2001**, *39*, 8–17.

508. Wang, X. *Increased Taxol Production in Taxus× Media through Metabolic Engineering Approaches*; Oklahoma State University: Stillwater, OK, USA, 2003.
509. Canales, N.A.; Hansen, T.N.G.; Cornett, C.; Walker, K.; Driver, F.; Antonelli, A.; Maldonado, C.; Nesbitt, M.; Barnes, C.J.; Rønsted, N. Historical chemical annotations of Cinchona bark collections are comparable to results from current day high-pressure liquid chromatography technologies. *J. Ethnopharmacol.* **2020**, *249*, 112375.
510. Dumas, E.; Giraudo, M.; Goujon, E.; Halma, M.; Knhili, E.; Stauffert, M.; Batisson, I.; Besse-Hoggan, P.; Bohatier, J.; Bouchard, P. Fate and ecotoxicological impact of new generation herbicides from the triketone family: An overview to assess the environmental risks. *J. Hazard. Mater.* **2017**, *325*, 136–156.
511. Miller, H.P.; Bonawitz, S.C.; Ostrovsky, O. The effects of delta-9-tetrahydrocannabinol (THC) on inflammation: A review. *Cell. Immunol.* **2020**, *352*, 104111.
512. Wong, J.C.M. Contribution of Intestinal Lymphatic Transport to the Antiproliferative Effect of delta-9-Tetrahydrocannabinol. Ph.D. Thesis, University of Nottingham, Nottingham, UK, 2017.
513. Ahn, Y.; Han, S.H.; Kim, M.G.; Hong, K.-B.; Kim, W.J.; Suh, H.J.; Jo, K. Anti-depressant effects of ethanol extract from Cannabis sativa (hemp) seed in chlorpromazine-induced Drosophila melanogaster depression model. *Pharm. Biol.* **2021**, *59*, 998–1007.
514. Bonini, S.A.; Premoli, M.; Tambaro, S.; Kumar, A.; Maccarinelli, G.; Memo, M.; Mastinu, A. Cannabis sativa: A comprehensive

ethnopharmacological review of a medicinal plant with a long history. *J. Ethnopharmacol.* **2018**, *227*, 300–315.

515. Cantele, C.; Bertolino, M.; Bakro, F.; Giordano, M.; Jędryczka, M.; Cardenia, V. Antioxidant effects of hemp (Cannabis sativa L.) inflorescence extract in stripped linseed oil. *Antioxidants* **2020**, *9*, 1131.
516. Mohammad, A.; Faruqi, F.B.; Mustafa, J. Edible compounds as antitumor agents Ali Mohammad1, Fauzia Bano Faruqi1 and Jamal Mustafa2. *Indian. J. Sci. Technol.* **2009**, *2*, 62–74.
517. Chaachouay, N.; Azeroual, A.; Bencherki, B.; Douira, A.; Zidane, L. Various Metabolites and or Bioactive Compounds from Vegetables, and Their Use Nanoparticles Synthesis, and Applications. In *Nanomaterials from Agricultural and Horticultural Products*; Husen, A., Ed.; Smart Nanomaterials Technology; Springer Nature: Singapore, 2023; pp. 187–209.
518. Grigoriev, O.V. Application of hempseed (*Cannabis sativa* L.) oil in the treatment of ear, nose and throat (ENT) disorders. *J. Ind. Hemp* **2002**, *7*, 5–15.
519. Havey, M.J. Onion: *Allium cepa* L. In *Genetic Improvement of Vegetable Crops*; Pergamon Press: Oxford, UK; New York, NY, USA, 1993; pp. 35–49.
520. Ashraf, R.; Khan, R.A.; Ashraf, I. Garlic (Allium sativum) supplementation with standard antidiabetic agent provides better diabetic control in type 2 diabetes patients. *Pak. J. Pharm. Sci.* **2011**, *24*, 565–570.
521. Rajput, H. Effects of Atropa belladonna as an anti-cholinergic. *Nat. Prod. Chem. Res.* **2013**, *1*, 104.

522. Imanshahidi, M.; Hosseinzadeh, H. Pharmacological and therapeutic effects of Berberis vulgaris and its active constituent, berberine. *Phytother. Res.* **2008**, *22*, 999–1012.
523. López, V.; Calvo, M.I. White tea (*Camellia sinensis* Kuntze) exerts neuroprotection against hydrogen peroxide-induced toxicity in PC12 cells. *Plant Foods Hum. Nutr.* **2011**, *66*, 22–26.
524. Zhao, D.; Hamilton, J.P.; Pham, G.M.; Crisovan, E.; Wiegert-Rininger, K.; Vaillancourt, B.; DellaPenna, D.; Buell, C.R. De novo genome assembly of Camptotheca acuminata, a natural source of the anti-cancer compound camptothecin. *GigaScience* **2017**, *6*, gix065.
525. Novak, M.; Salemink, C.A.; Khan, I. Biological activity of the alkaloids of Erythroxylum coca and Erythroxylum novogranatense. *J. Ethnopharmacol.* **1984**, *10*, 261–274.
526. Singh, H.P.; Utreja, P.; Tiwary, A.K.; Jain, S. Elastic liposomal formulation for sustained delivery of colchicine: In vitro characterization and in vivo evaluation of anti-gout activity. *AAPS J.* **2009**, *11*, 54–64.
527. Morimoto, M.; Tatsumi, K.; Yuui, K.; Terazawa, I.; Kudo, R.; Kasuda, S. Convallatoxin, the primary cardiac glycoside in lily of the valley (Convallaria majalis), induces tissue factor expression in endothelial cells. *Vet. Med. Sci.* **2021**, *7*, 2440–2444.
528. Bhusare, B.P.; John, C.K.; Bhatt, V.P.; Nikam, T.D. In Vitro propagation of Digitalis lanata Ehrh. through direct shoot regeneration—A source of cardiotonic glycosides. *Ind. Crops Prod.* **2018**, *121*, 313–319.
529. Kvasnička, F.; Bıba, B.; Ševčík, R.; Voldřich, M.; Kratka, J. Analysis of the active components of silymarin. *J. Chromatogr. A* **2003**, *990*, 239–245.

530. Haley, T.J. Metabolism and pharmacokinetics of theophylline in human neonates, children, and adults. *Drug Metab. Rev.* **1983**, *14*, 295–335.

About Authors

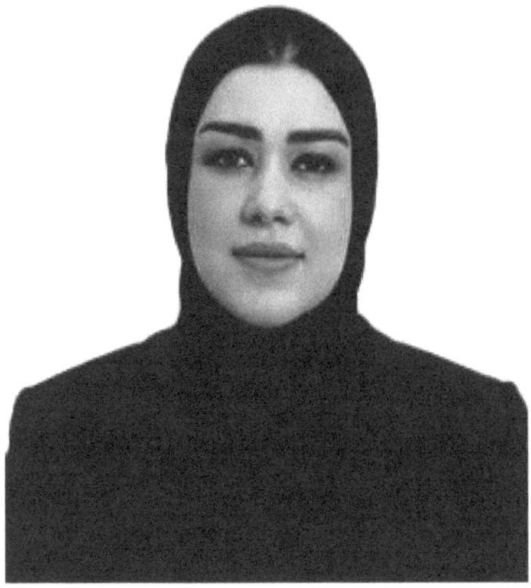

Assist. Prof. Dr. Widad A. Abd Al-Behadili

Department of Pharmacognosy and Medicinal Plants, College of Pharmacy, University of Misan, Maysan, Iraq.

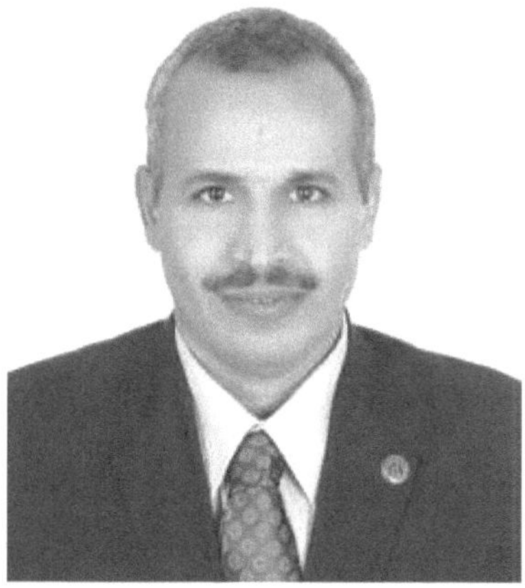

Prof. Dr. Mohamed Abdel-Raheem Ali Abdel-Raheem

Professor of Biological Control

Pests & Plant Protection Department

Agricultural and Biological Research Institute

National Research Centre.

Prof. Dr. Mohamed Abdel-Raheem Ali Abdel-Raheem, Prof. of Entomology (Biological Control), Pests & Plant Protection Department, Agricultural and Biological Research Institute, National Research Centre, Cairo, Egypt. Published publications (329) papers (89), Books and Book chapters (240), Edited books (8), (Scopus) h-index (12), Citations (343), (Google Scholar) h-index (21) , Citations (1215), (Web of Science) Publications (29), h-index (11), Citations (315), Research Gate, h-index (15), Citations (734), Reviewers in International Journals (159), Reviewed articles in Biological Control (1087), Editor in Chief in Journal (7), Assistant Editor (1), Associated Editor in Chief in Journal (7), Editorial board in Journals (42), Advisory board (1), conference Attended (27), workshop Attended (313), Symposium Attended (179), Forum Attended (4), Prize (4), Attended Others (30), Projects As PI and member (20), Training courses For Agric. Engineering (61), Training courses For Students of University (12), attending Trainees courses (19), TV, Radio & Newspaper (39), Supervisor on Ms.C. thesis (3), Supervisor on Ph.D. thesis (1), Committee Ph.D. Thesis in Egypt (2), and member in scientific Foundation (14), Giving International lectures (4), Promotion Committee Prof. international (2), Committee Ph.D. thesis international (1).

National Research Centre. 33rd ElBohouth St., Dokki, Cairo, Egypt.

Email Address: abdelraheem_nrc@hotmail.com, ma.abdel-raheem@nrc.sci.eg, abdelraheem_nrc@yahoo.com, profmohamedabdelraheem@gmail.com, abdelraheem196942@gmail.com, mabdelraheem69@gmail.com, mabdelraheem69@yahoo.com.

Mobile Phone: (+2) 01155527583 – (+2) 01009580797

Scopus Author ID : 55220661700

https://www.scopus.com/authid/detail.uri?authorId=55220661700

http://scholar.google.com/citations?hl=en&user=gBtssEgAAAAJ

https://orcid.org/my-orcid?orcid=0000-0001-9240-064X

https://www.webofscience.com/wos/author/searchAbdel-Raheem, Mohamed Abdel-Raheem Ali - Web of Science Core Collection

https://www.researchgate.net/profile/Mohamed_Abdel-Raheem4/publications?sorting=recentlyAdded

http://livedna.org/20.16018

http://www.resarcherid.com/rid/R-6264-2017

https://www.webofscience.com/wos/author/record/R-6264-2017

https://www.facebook.com/share/p/1Piu6xyFmN/

- TV, Radio & Newspaper links

1. https://www.youtube.com/attribution_link?a=NsH2xGv9mY8&u=%2Fwatch%3Fv%3Dsb46rBG8-Mc%26feature%3Dshare
2. https://youtu.be/Ub8djW0tggo
3. https://m.facebook.com/story.php?story_fbid=492907069288338&id=100076011247165
4. https://youtu.be/dOujUAZmTdw
5. https://m.facebook.com/story.php?story_fbid=492907069288338&id=100076011247165
6. https://fb.watch/gPGrDuzZFX/
7. https://www.youtube.com/watch?si=4UfyQaeHVLPiVR5J&v=nXV4NT-no7o&feature=youtu.be
8. https://www.youtube.com/watch?v=sRH44W6TbcQ
9. https://youtu.be/uq9Qj3AEBHk?si=ymaX06huG2AXJESu
10. https://www.facebook.com/share/v/Qg5s6HW3hD8PLBzp/?mibextid=xfxF2i

11. https://el-yom.com/news/archives/1092767
12. https://el-yomnews.com/?p=1156515
13. https://el-yomnews.com/%D8%A7%D9%84%D8%AF%D9%83%D8%AA%D9%88%D8%B1-%D8%B9%D8%A8%D8%AF%D8%A7%D9%84%D8%B1%D8%AD%D9%8A%D9%85-%D9%85%D8%AD%D9%85%D8%AF-%D8%B9%D9%84%D9%8A-%D9%8A%D8%AA%D8%AD%D8%AF%D8%AB-%D9%84%D9%84%D9%84/
14. https://el-yomnews.com/?p=1179515
15. https://www.facebook.com/share/v/4MM85wKRPxsYLqTr/
16. http://https//el-yomnews.com/%D8%A7%D9%84%D8%AD%D8%B4%D8%B1%D8%A7%D8%AA-%D9%81%D9%8A-%D8%AE%D8%AF%D9%85%D8%A9-%D8%A7%D9%84%D8%B9%D8%AF%D8%A7%D9%84%D8%A9-%D9%85%D8%AD%D8%A7%D8%B6%D8%B1%D8%A9-%D8%AA%D9%83%D8%B4%D9%81-%D8%AF%D9%88/
17. https://youtube.com/watch?v=F21ziQxdeco&si=LvSUixmnSg4JM1zK
18. https://youtu.be/F21ziQxdeco?si=jyAwbU8dVwkYzRH4
19- https://el-yomnews.com/المكافحة-الحيوية-بالفطريات-حلول-مبتك/
20- https://el-yomnews.com/archives/1296404
21- https://www.facebook.com/share/p/1AC25ue5XG/
22- https://youtu.be/7VItE5kON2g?si=9rMWMUSGk8Csgjfn
23- https://www.youtube.com/watch?v=G9nXA7Q9C60
24- https://www.youtube.com/watch?v=7VItE5kON2g

25- https://el-yomnews.com/archives/1347977

26- https://youtu.be/x9N58DakONg?si=Uh0HbpQsiDRpIGMl

27- https://youtu.be/PfuQy-Zkq3s?si=GtRRxy9XtTW-YgF3

28- https://youtu.be/Vo1NqVmPxMU?si=vJxt4YyhzqJL9hR4

29- https://youtu.be/pqo5F-cbGSc?si=J_B9Dv05bfX5P-7O

TV and Radio

1- Filming in the program (Meeting the Scientists) - Al-Manara Channel, entitled Biological Control of Insect Pests, on 7/2/2013.

2- Filming in the program (Friends of Al-Manara) - Al-Manara Channel, February 2014.

3- A recording of an interview with the program (From the Secrets of the Universe and Life) Radio Sawt Al-Arab, Cairo on 4/26/2015.

4- Filming in the program (Idea for a bobbin) - Nile Cultural Channel under the title "Using entomopathogenic fungi and plant extracts in combating insect pests that infect sugar crops in Egypt" on 11/1/2015.

5- Filming on (This Morning) program - Nile News Channel under the title: Submitting the specifications for the reclamation of one and a half million feddans as a first stage of the reclamation of 4 million feddans on 11/15/2015. https://www.youtube.com/attribution_link?a=NsH2xGv9mY8&u=%2Fwatch%3Fv%3Dsb46rBG8-Mc%26feature%3Dshare

6- Registration in the program (Our Life Between Our Hands) for North Upper Egypt Radio and Radio, presented by Dr. Essam Fathy, 3 episodes, on 11-29-

2021, and it will be broadcast on Saturday and Wednesday at 3:30 pm in January 2022

7- Registration in the program (Our Life Between Our Hands) for North Upper Egypt Radio and Radio, presented by Dr. Essam Fathy, 3 episodes, on 11-29-2021, and it will be broadcast on Saturday and Wednesday at 3:30 pm in January 2022
8- Registration in the program (Our Life Between Our Hands) for North Upper Egypt Radio and Radio, presented by Dr. Essam Fathy, 3 episodes, on 11-29-2021, and it will be broadcast on Saturday and Wednesday at 3:30 pm in January 2022
9- Registration in "Our Green Land" program for North Upper Egypt Radio and Radio, presented by Dr. Essam Fathy, 3 episodes, on 11-2021-2021, to be broadcast in January 2022
10- Registration in "Our Green Land" program for North Upper Egypt Radio and Radio, presented by Dr. Essam Fathy, 3 episodes, on 11-2021-2021, to be broadcast in January 2022
11- Registration in "Our Green Land" program for North Upper Egypt Radio and Radio, presented by Dr. Essam Fathy, 3 episodes, on 11-2021-2021, to be broadcast in January 2022
12- Filming in the program (Egypt is Beautiful) - the second Egyptian Nile Channel, under the title: Climate Changes on November 6, 2022. https://youtu.be/dOujUAZmTdw
13- Registration in "Our Green Land" program for North Upper Egypt Radio and Radio, presented by Dr. Essam Fathy, 3 episodes, on 11-2021-2021, to be broadcast in January 2022

14- Filming in the program (Egypt and Climate Summit) - Delta Satellite Channel under the title: Climate Cop 27 on 13/11/2022 https://youtu.be/Ub8djW0tggo

15- Filming in (Egypt) - Sohag, Coral Times Hotel, under the title: Climate Change, Cop 27, dated 11/15/2022, the journalist Shorouk Abdullah https://m.facebook.com/story.php?story_fbid=492907069288338&id=100076011247165

16- Filming in (Feed and Benefit) - Coral Hotel in Sohag under the title: Climate Cop 27 on 11/15/2022, journalist Ahmed Tarboush https://fb.watch/gPGrDuzZFX/

17- An intervention in the plant clinic program on insect-pathogenic fungi in Egypt's agricultural farms on Thursday 29/2/2024.
https://www.youtube.com/watch?si=4UfyQaeHVLPiVR5J&v=nXV4NT-no7o&feature=youtu.be

18- Filming in the plant clinic program on the Misr Agricultural Channel about insect-pathogenic fungi on Sunday 3-3-2024
https://www.youtube.com/watch?v=sRH44W6TbcQ

19- Filming in the plant clinic program at the Misr Agricultural Channel, early prediction of the red palm weevil and modern methods of combating it, on Thursday 25/4/2024.
https://youtu.be/uq9Qj3AEBHk?si=ymaX06huG2AXJESu

20- Filming in the Green Planet program on the Egyptian Channel 2 (Biological Control) on Sunday 7/6/2024
https://www.facebook.com/watch/?v=981454710052376

21- A press interview in Al-Youm newspaper with journalist Mr. Imad Naseer on 7-30-2024. https://el-yom.com/news/archives/1092767
https://el-yomnews.com/

22- https://el-yomnews.com/?p=1156515
23- https://el-yomnews.com/%D8%A7%D9%84%D8%AF%D9%83%D8%AA%D9%88%D8%B1-%D8%B9%D8%A8%D8%AF%D8%A7%D9%84%D8%B1%D8%AD%D9%8A%D9%85-%D9%85%D8%AD%D9%85%D8%AF-%D8%B9%D9%84%D9%8A-%D9%8A%D8%AA%D8%AD%D8%AF%D8%AB-%D9%84-%D9%84%D9%84/
24- https://el-yomnews.com/?p=1179515
25- https://www.facebook.com/share/v/4MM85wKRPxsYLqTr/
26- Insects in the Service of Justice: A Lecture Explaining the Role of Forensic Entomology in Investigating Crimes
https://el-yomnews.com/archives/1243894
27- Human health is at risk. An investigation reveals the secrets of pesticide-contaminated agriculture.
https://el-yomnews.com/archives/1296404
28- https://www.facebook.com/share/p/1AC25ue5XG/
The Green Planet Program (Beneficial Insects and Their Role in the Environment) on 5/23/2025 on the Egyptian Channel 2
29- https://youtu.be/7VItE5kON2g?si=9rMWMUSGk8Csgjfn
30- https://www.youtube.com/watch?v=G9nXA7Q9C60
31- https://www.youtube.com/watch?v=7VItE5kON2g
32- https://el-yomnews.com/archives/1347977
33- https://youtu.be/x9N58DakONg?si=Uh0HbpQsiDRpIGMl
34- https://youtu.be/PfuQy-Zkq3s?si=GtRRxy9XtTW-YgF3

35- https://youtu.be/Vo1NqVmPxMU?si=vJxt4YyhzqJL9hR4

36- https://youtu.be/pqo5F-cbGSc?si=J_B9Dv05bfX5P-7O

FSC
www.fsc.org
MIX
Papier | Fördert gute Waldnutzung
FSC® C083411

Kolibri 360 GmbH
Ferdinand-Jühlke-Straße 7
99095 Erfurt, Deutschland
produktsicherheit@kolibri360.de

Druck:
CPI Druckdienstleistungen GmbH
im Auftrag der
Kolibri 360 GmbH
Ferdinand-Jühlke-Str. 7
99095 Erfurt